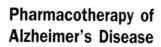

Pharmacotherapy of
Alzheimer's Disease

Pharmacotherapy of Alzheimer's Disease

Edited by

Serge Gauthier MD FRCP(C)
McGill Center for Studies in Aging
Douglas Hospital
Verdun PQ
Canada

Foreword by

Claudio Cuello MD
Chair
Department of Pharmacology and Therapeutics
McGill University
Montreal PQ
Canada

MARTIN DUNITZ

© Martin Dunitz Ltd 1998

First published in the United Kingdom in 1998 by
Martin Dunitz Ltd
The Livery House
7-9 Pratt Street
London NW1 0AE

A CIP catalogue record for this book is available from the British Library

ISBN 1-85317-583-8

Distributed in the USA, Canada and Brazil
by
Blackwell Science Inc
Commerce Place
350 Main Street
Malden
MA 02148-5018
USA
Tel: 1-800-215-1000

Composition by Scribe Design, Gillingham, Kent
Printed and bound in Italy

This book is dedicated to the memory of Dr Luigi Amaducci, a gentleman and true scientist, whose contribution to the understanding of the etiology and treatment of Alzheimer's disease will have a lasting impact on patients worldwide.

Merci Luigi et au revoir

Serge Gauthier
April 1998

Contents

Contributors

†Luigi Amaducci MD
Director, Department of Neurological Psychiatric
Sciences, University of Florence, 50134 Florence, Italy.

François Boller MD
Professor, Service de Gérontologie, Hôpital Broca-CHU
Cochin-Université Paris V, 75013 Paris; and U324
INSERM, 75014 Paris, France.

Laura Bracco MD
Professor, Department of Neurological Psychiatric
Sciences, University of Florence, 50134 Florence, Italy.

Henry Brodaty MB BS (SYD) MD (NSW) FRACP
Professor of Psychogeriatrics, School of Psychiatry,
University of New South Wales and Director,
Academic Department of Psychogeriatrics, Prince
Henry Hospital, Little Bay NSW 2036, Australia.

Claudio Cuello MD DSc FRSC
Chair, Department of Pharmacology and Therapeutics,
McGill University, Montreal PQ, Canada H3G 1Y6.

† Deceased

Albert Enz Ing.chem.
Senior Scientist and Biochemist, Novartis Pharma Inc. CH-4002 Basel, Switzerland.

Sanford I Finkel MD
Professor, Department of Psychiatry, Northwestern University, Chicago, IL 60611, USA.

Françoise Forette MD
Service de Gérontologie, Hôpital Broca-CHU Cochin-Université Paris V, 75013 Paris; and U324 INSERM, 75014 Paris, France.

Serge Gauthier MD FRCP (C)
Professor, Department of Neurology and Neurosurgery, Psychiatry, Medicine, McGill University, The McGill Centre for Studies in Aging, Douglas Hospital, Verdun PQ, Canada H4H 1R3.

Ezio Giacobini MD
Adjunct Professor, Institutions Universitaires de Gériatrie de Genève, 1226 Thonex-Genève Switzerland.

Michael Grundman MD MPH
Associate Clinical Professor of Neurosciences, University of California at San Diego, La Jolla CA 92093-0949, USA.

Bernie J O'Brien PhD
Associate Professor, Department of Clinical Epidemiology and Biostatics, McMaster University; and Centre for the Evaluation of Medicines, St Joseph's Hospital, Hamilton ON, Canada L8N 4A6.

Michel Panisset MD
Asistant Professor, Department of Neurology and Neurosurgery, McGill University, Centre McGill d'études sur le vieillissement, Hôpital Douglas, Verdun PQ, Canada H4H 1R3.

Carolina Piccini MD
Neurologist, Department of Neurological Psychiatric
Sciences, University of Florence, 50134 Florence,
Italy.

Judes Poirier PhD
The McGill Centre for Studies in Aging, Douglas
Hospital, Verdun PQ, Canada H4H 1R3.

Stephen G Post PhD
Professor, Case Western Reserve University, School
of Medicine, Cleveland OH 44106-4976,
USA.

Leon J Thal MD
Professor and Chair, Department of Neurosciences,
University of California at San Diego, La Jolla CA
92093-0624, USA.

Peter J Whitehouse MD PhD
Professor, University of Cleveland, University
Alzheimer Center, Cleveland OH 44120-1013,
USA.

Foreword

Claudio Cuello

It is with great pleasure that I write a few lines as foreword to this much-needed volume, *'Pharmacotherapy of Alzheimer's Disease'*. At present, the field of Alzheimer's disease research is plagued by an abundance of information of varied relevance to our understanding of the disease and the therapeutics of afflicted individuals, now and in the future. Intense research in the field, both basic and clinical, has created considerable confusion and many misconceptions. The fact that there are no universal rules as to how clinical trials should be conceived and evaluated adds to the bewilderment of clinicians and interested scientists, and of caregivers alike. The great merit of this book is the comprehensive framework it offers for the evaluation of seemingly contradictory information.

In this book, Serge Gauthier invited a number of leading specialists to write on a broad range of fundamental issues in Alzheimer's disease, from the recent history of Alzheimer therapy to the social and ethical consequences of current and future therapeutics. The chapters maintain a uniformly concise and straightforward style that will be much appreciated by readers. And just who will read this book? I foresee that the main group will be clinicians confronting the challenges posed by the idiosyncratic responses of their patients to the therapies currently available. Several chapters in this book will prove useful to them by shedding light on why a patient responds (or does not) to therapy with the current generation of acetyl cholinesterase inhibitors, and also by highlighting potential alternative therapies.

'Pharmacotherapy of Alzheimer's Disease' has the further merit of examining the main medical cultures which exist internationally, explaining how these condition the way in which clinical trials are conceived and evaluated, and how drugs are approved and accepted as viable therapeutics by their respective medical communities, patients and caregivers. It also offers a useful review of the significance of the diverse scores and scales used to assess cognitive deficits and deterioration marking progression of the disease. The reader should not expect to find here an instruction manual for their

use, but rather a guide as to how and when these tools should be applied.

Clearly, nowadays, the use of anti-cholinesterases is the main pharmacological weapon in Alzheimer's disease therapy. The scientific and historical reasons for this are clearly delineated in a couple of chapters, with abundant cross references being provided in others. While these drugs have not realized the impact of L-DOPA therapy in Parkinson's disease, it is becoming increasingly clear that they will play an important role in contemporary Alzheimer's disease therapeutics. The limitations of this therapy, as well as its medical, social, and ethical advantages and disadvantages are extensively and most lucidly discussed.

Gauthier and his team do not deal at length with possible future therapeutic avenues. Rather, various possibilities are mentioned in a number of chapters and a comprehensive summary is provided at the conclusion. The tone is characteristically cautious, with none of the hyperbole that, unfortunately, we have become accustomed to receive from the modern media. Nevertheless, we are left with a positive and optimistic feeling that 'something' is coming. This is not an entirely unrealistic scenario, since much of the necessary molecular neuropathology has been elucidated in the past few decades, and new animal models, which more closely replicate the disease state, are becoming increasingly available for preclinical explorations with a new generation of drugs. Indeed, we expect that the next decade will see important new therapeutic avenues for the management of Alzheimer's disease.

In closing, I only hope that any future edition of the '*Pharmacotherapy of Alzheimer's Disease*' will address these new developments with the same helpful and clear style that has been applied in this edition. The personal charisma of Serge Gauthier has undoubtedly helped to attract such a distinguished list of authors. Their colleagues in the basic and clinical sciences, as well as the general public, should be grateful for their efforts.

Claudio Cuello MD
Montreal, April 1998

Introduction

Serge Gauthier

As we begin 1998, we are at a turning point in the history of the pharmacotherapy of Alzheimer's disease (AD), with widely available cholinesterase inhibitors such as tacrine, donepezil and rivastigmime, soon to be followed by metrifonate. These agents have been developed over the last 12 years as substitution therapy for the central cholinergic deficit associated with AD, and help symptoms in early to intermediate stages in many patients. Other types of symptomatic drugs are under study or regulatory review, including muscarinic agonists and propentofylline. Furthermore, a number of drugs aiming at disease stabilization are under study, on the basis of selected etiology-driven hypotheses.

The authors of this book felt that it was timely to step back and assess what has been achieved in terms of trial designs and outcome variables for the randomized clinical trials, prior to the publications in peer-reviewed journals of the bulk of phase III data. We hope that this component of the book will facilitate the reading and interpretation of the relevant literature. Regulatory, ethical and pharmacoeconomic considerations are also important in the overall process of AD drug development, and are discussed in depth.

We wanted to facilitate the use of AD-specific drugs by proposing guidelines based on the available, albeit limited, experience outside of randomized clinical trials. The point of view of families and caregivers is clearly expressed. We hope that clinicians of all disciplines caring for persons with AD will find in these pages cause for optimism.

Drug development in Alzheimer's disease: a review of its history and a preview of its future

Françoise Forette and François Boller

1

Introduction

A recent opinion poll has shown that among French women over 35, Alzheimer's disease (AD) is the most feared of all medical conditions.[1] What are the reasons for such a high level of concern? After all, the disease in its definite or probable form is relatively uncommon, since its prevalence is less than 5% in subjects over 65. The data provided by the PAQUID study suggest that around 350 000 persons are affected in France.[2,3] However, the late onset of this disease, which has now become well known to the public, induces a deep fear that minor problems with memory and other commonly occurring temporary cognitive lapses may represent the prodromes of AD. In addition, demographic and epidemiological data point to an enormous increase in the aging population in both developed and developing countries.[4] Extrapolations based on population studies suggest that by the year 2000 there will be several millions of demented patients in North America[5,6] and in Europe.[7] It is also true that, until recently, the disease was perceived as devastating because of its irreversible progression towards intellectual and physical deterioration, the total absence of curative and preventive therapy and the poor medico-social support available in most countries.

In the past 10 years or so, however, there have been several advances in the therapy of AD, and some medications are already available to produce some symptomatic improvements in many patients. These medications have clear limitations in terms of time and efficacy, but recent data on the genetics and the molecular biology of AD should provide the premises for more rational and physiopathologically oriented treatments of the disease in the not so distant future.[8]

Substitution therapies

Cholinergic treatments

In recent years, there has been a very large number of therapeutic trials addressing AD and related disorders. Among them, those involving cholinergic agents are of particular interest, because they have been the first to

lead to drugs officially recognized for the treatment of AD. They are all based on the so-called cholinergic theory.

This theory is based on the assumption that acetylcholine (ACh) metabolism plays an important role in memory processes. Furthermore, according to this theory, the deterioration of memory and other cognitive functions in AD is directly related to degeneration of cerebral presynaptic cholinergic neurons. This theory is usually attributed to independent observations by Bowen et al[9] and by Davies and Maloney[10] that choline acetyltransferase (CAT) is frequently deficient in autopsy material from patients with AD, a finding often replicated in later years. It was also found that changes in the cholinergic system correlate with the severity of dementia.[11] These findings led subsequent researchers to trace the neurochemical changes to malfunction and destruction of cholinergic neurons in the basal nucleus of Meynert,[12,13] a structure known to be of particular importance in the cholinergic system of animals and humans.[14]

Long before that, however, the effect on memory of atropine and other drugs related to ACh metabolism had been noted. As far back as 1906 (about the time when Alzheimer presented his famous case),[15] it was found that a combination of a central anticholinergic and sedatives causes a change in mental status called 'twilight sleep'.[16] This combination of drugs was used occasionally, especially in the 1950s and 1960s, to produce altered consciousness in mothers during childbirth. In 1974, Drachman and Leavitt[17] found that scopolamine induces a memory disorder in normal volunteers which affects learning abilities but not the capacity to recall previously learned material. Comparisons of the memory and cognitive deficits induced by scopolamine with the performance of aged subjects revealed a marked similarity of pattern. Therefore, it can be argued that this paper[17] was the first to postulate a role for the cholinergic system in relation to memory and aging.

Even though it has been known for years that other neurotransmitters are involved in AD, the cholinergic theory soon raised hope that replacement or at least increased availability of ACh might improve memory in the aged and in patients affected by AD, analogously to the effect of L-DOPA in Parkinson' disease. On the basis of the cholinergic theory, four potential pharmacological strategies are available as follows:

Use of ACh precursors

This approach has been pursued mainly by providing exogenous choline[18] or phosphatidylcholine (lecithin).[19] Unfortunately the great majority of studies using this method have failed to produce positive results (see Becker and Giacobini[20] for a review).

ACh releasers

This class of drugs includes pyridine derivatives such as 4-aminopyridine and 3,4-diaminopyridine. They have been tried with limited success in animals and, in a few cases, in humans.[21] Other compounds such as phosphatidylserine, which may increase synthesis and release of ACh, have only been tried to a limited extent in humans.

Direct-acting ACh agonists

The advantage of this class of drugs is that they act on postsynaptic cholinergic (muscarinic) receptors which appear to be relatively unaffected in AD. Most of them, however, are either very short-acting or do not cross the blood–brain barrier. Arecoline given by multiple intravenous infusions has been shown to have some slight positive effects,[22] but this form of administration is obviously impractical. In 1984, Harbaugh et al[23] reported some improvement (noticed by families blind to the treatment) in patients with intra-ventricular administration of bethane-chol, but a later multicentre trial[23,24] proved disappointing.

Some therapeutic trials have involved non-muscarinic receptors known to be affected in AD and, specifically, nicotinic receptors. It is well known that nicotine affects attention, memory and rapid information encoding in humans.[25] It has been suggested that nicotinic agonists have the potential to increase both cholinergic and dopamin-ergic transmission.[26]

Cholinesterase inhibitors

This approach was introduced in the late 1970s[27] and is the only 'cholinergic strategy' for which some success has been consistently demonstrated. Because physostigmine is relatively safe, crosses the blood–brain barrier easily and is available in oral form (even though its absorption is poor),[28] many researchers have used it. In their review, Becker and Giacobini[20] found that 20 of 31 studies reported some improvement in memory when physostigmine was used. In most cases, however (see, for example, Beuer et al[29]), improvements

were modest and short-lived even when physostigmine was combined with ACh precursors such as lecithine.[30] Tacrine was introduced because it was felt to be less potent but a longer-acting centrally active cholinesterase inhibitor than physostigmine.

History of THA

9-Amino-1,2,3,4-tetrahydroxyacridine (THA) was first synthesized in 1945 by Albert et al[31] who were investigating the relationship between the various structures of acridine antiseptics and their action. In a paper reviewing the history of THA, Thornton and Gershon[32] showed that subsequently the drug had many uses, including counteracting some of the effects of psychotomimetic drugs. It was used in the UK and in Australia mainly by anaesthesiologists to counteract the respiratory depression produced by morphine without affecting its analgesic effect. It was also used in combination with curare. It was withdrawn from the market in the UK in 1982, apparently because it was used very little, since other more effec-tive anti-curare agents were available.

Beside its anticholinesterase activity and its being a partial agonist of morphine, THA probably has other pharmacological actions.[32] These include an effect on excitatory amino acids such as aspartate and glutamate, blockage of channels associated with monovalent cations, particularly potassium,[33] and action on components of the monaminergic system.[34] In addition, it prolongs the action of suxamethonium and inhibits monoamine oxidase and cyclic AMP.

THA was first used in AD in the early 1980s,[35,36] with what were considered 'modest results'. However, in an article published by the prestigious *New England Journal of Medicine* in November 1986,[37] Summers et al reported having treated 17 patients with the diagnosis of AD, 12 of whom had entered a phase of long-term administration of oral THA. The degree of improvement, they wrote, 'had often been dramatic'. At least some improvement was observed in all subjects, and 'no serious side effects attributable to THA had been observed'.

Several subsequent studies provided results that were sometimes equivocal. The 'final' word was given only recently, thanks to the results of trials of larger sample size. Two studies conducted respectively in North America and in France[38,39] found a significant clinical benefit on the ADAS-Cog and the ADAS-Total, less so on the IADL and the 'Progressive Deterioration Scale', and not on the 'Clinical Global Impression' (CGI). The study by Knapp et al[40] demonstrated dose-related clinical efficacy, as judged on the ADAS-Cog, the Clinician Based Impression of Change (CIBI) and the Final Comprehensive Consensus Assessment (FCCA).

Tacrine, unfortunately, is not without side-effects, which include hepatotoxicity and cholinergic peripheral effects such as nausea and diarrhoea; in addition, it requires a four-times-a-day administration and an extended titration. In spite of these problems, the drug was approved by the FDA in the USA in 1995 and later on in France and in many other countries. Since that time, a report has shown a delay in the institutionalization of patients who tolerate the drug at therapeutic doses.[41]

Other cholinergic agents

The 'tacrine story' has prompted the development of other drugs. The following are now or are soon going to be on the market:

- Donepezil or E2020, known commercially as Aricept. E2020 is a piperidine cholinesterase inhibitor (ChEI) which is structurally distinct from other compounds presently under study for treatment of Alzheimer's disease. It has been studied extensively in animals.[42] Phase III studies performed in the USA have shown good efficacy and tolerability in patients with mild to moderate AD.[43] The drug is now available in the USA, Canada and many other countries.

- ENA 713 (Exelon, Sandoz) is a central nervous system (CNS)-selective, pseudoirreversible ChEI also shows brain region selectivity. It is not metabolized by the hepatic microsomal system. Its duration of cholinesterase inhibition is 10 h. Phase II trials using doses of 6–12 mg/day have suggested efficacy and reasonably low levels of side-effects. Phase III trials suggest an efficacy comparable to that of other, newer ChEIs.[44] The drug has recently been released in Switzerland.

- Metrifonate is an organophosphate which, through the action of its metabolite dichlorvinyl dimethyl phosphate (DDVP or dichlorvos), produces an irreversible cholinesterase enzyme inhibition and increases local cerebral glucose utilization in young and aged rats.[45] One study[46] showed a mean of 52.3% decrease in red blood cell acetyl-cholinesterase activity. During up to 18 months of subsequent open metrifonate treatment, there was a deterioration of 1.68 points per year in Minimum Mental State Examination (MMSE) performance. Adverse effects were uncommon and did not require adjustment of the dose of metrifonate or discontinuation of treatment. The drug is under regulatory review in Europe and North America.

There are many other cholinergic agents currently under development. A partial list[47] includes the following.

- Cholinesterase inhibitors:
  Eptastigmine (Mediolanum)
  Sustained-release physostigmine (Synapton, Forest)
  Huperzine (Chinese Academy of Science)
  NX-066 (Astra Arcus)
  KA-672 (Schwabe)
  Galanthamine (Janssen)
- Cholinergic receptor agents:
  Milameline (Warner–Lambert)
  AF102B (Forest/Snow Brand Products)
  SB202026 (SmithKline Beecham)

Xanomeline (Lilly)
ENS 163 (Sandoz)
Talsaclidine (Boehringer-Ingelheim)
LU 25109 (Lundbeck)
• Indirect cholinergic enhancers:
ABT 418 (Abbott)
ABT 089 (Abbott)

Other replacement treatments

As mentioned above, AD affects several neurotransmitter systems. This has been the rationale for several therapeutic trials involving systems other than the cholinergic one.[48]

Even though the adrenergic system is known to be implicated in memory storage, recall and selective attention, the efficacy of biogenic amines has never been proven: trials with L-DOPA, amantadine, bromocriptine and pirebidil have given contradictory, but on the whole negative, results.[49] Similarly, despite the known involvement of the serotonergic system, block of 5-HT recapture has been without effect on cognition.

Neuropeptides have been studied extensively. Despite the known somatostatinergic deficit,[50] somatostatin analogues have not shown impressive results. This applies also to vasopressin analogues, to adrenocorticotrophic hormone (ACTH) and to other neuropeptides such as thyrotropine releasing hormone (TRH), vasoactive intestinal peptide (VIP) and neuropeptide Y. Excitatory amino acids such as glutamate or aspartate are implicated in synaptic mechanisms and play a major role in the potentiation of neurotransmission. The N-methyl D aspartate (NMDA) and aminohydroxy-5-methyl-4-isoazoproprionate (AMPA) receptors which are implicated in memory mechanisms have been the subject of recent research,[51] but the therapeutic trials have not yet produced practical results.

Clinical trials targeting neurotransmitters with complementary and potentiating action should be encouraged.

Despite their limitations, replacement therapies must be given credit for having taken AD out of the group of diseases totally inaccessible to pharmacological treatment. Clearly, however, they cannot durably modify the course of the disease, even less prevent it. Therapies of the future must therefore be based on an aetiological approach.

Aetiological approaches: therapies for the future

There is general agreement that AD is highly heterogeneous and that several different processes may lead to beta-amyloid deposits and neuronal loss (for review see Boller et al[52] and Shvaloff et al[53]). It is natural, therefore, that some therapeutic trials have been based on these processes, whether definite or only hypothetical.

Immunological theory

There are some data in favour of an immunological hyperreactivity in AD. These include microglial reaction around the senile plaques (SPs), astrocytosis, and production of inflammatory cytokines, some of which (interleukin-1 and interleukin-6) are said to increase the synthesis of a precursor of the amyloid protein.[54] Several studies have shown a reverse correlation between the occurrence of AD[55] or cognitive deterioration[56] and use of nonsteroidal anti-inflammatory agents. A therapeutic trial using indomethacin is in favour of this hypothesis.[57]

Neuroprotection: calcium channel blockers

The limited effect of substitution treatments may perhaps be explained by neuronal death. Calcium channel blockers might have a neuroprotective role by opposing intracellular influx of

calcium responsible for enzymatic activation and cell destruction. Several therapeutic trials used nimodipine to confirm the results of a short study which showed that this treatment tends to slow the rate of deterioration.[58]

Nerve growth factors

It has been known for some time that nerve growth factor (NGF) may have a trophic action at the level of nerve cells and particularly of cholinergic neurons. It is therefore natural to explore the possible therapeutic action of NGF, even though NGF decrease has not been postulated as an aetiological factor in AD. The future of NGF supplementation is, however, quite uncertain because of doubts concerning its efficacy, difficulty of delivery to the CNS and possible long-term toxicity.

One reason for concern is that NGF might cause an anarchic growth of neuritic connections with the potential to disrupt the existing neural network. It has also been suggested that NGF might potentiate the neurotoxic actions of the beta-amyloid protein. Finally, NGF does not cross the blood–brain barrier. The Swedish team that first applied this technique to humans used an intraventricular pump, and obtained only very limited clinical results.[59] The use of genetic engineering to produce subunits of human NGF able to cross the barrier and the development of molecules able to potentiate NGF activity may lead to better clinical results.[60] Research also involves several additional trophic factors, such as brain-derived neurotrophic factor (BDNF), ciliary neurotrophic factor (CNF), basic fibroblast growth factor (bFGF) and insulin-like growth factor (IGF-I).[61]

Agents acting on the amyloid protein

The neurotoxic role of A4 amyloid protein is now widely accepted. Yankner et al have shown that beta-amyloid plays two roles, toxic and neurotrophic, according to its concentration and the stage of neuronal development.[62] Also important is the observation of an inhibitory effect of some substances (neuropeptides) on the amyloid toxicity. Should these data apply to the living human brain, they might lead to the development of drugs able to 'disarm' the protein at the very beginning of the pathological process.

The production and the deposit of amyloid beta A4 by abnormal cleavage of the precursor amyloid precursor protein (APP) seems to be the principal element of the pathological process which in turn is the final common pathway of many potential mechanisms.[63]

The logical therapeutic approach is to attempt to intervene in the production, the deposit or the neurotoxiciy of the protein at the earliest possible stage of the disease in subjects at risk. Several directions are being pursued. They include the inhibition of the proteolytic enzymes capable of splitting the APP in an inappropriate or excessive fashion. The goal would be to inhibit beta or gamma secretases in favour of alpha secretases which allow the production of soluble non-amyloidogenic proteins, the inhibition of neurotoxicity, the reduction APP synthesis, the inhibition of the inflammatory reaction at the level of SPs, and the prevention or slowing down of polymerization of soluble proteins into amyloid fibrils.[64,65]

Genetic predisposition and treatment

In the last 10 years, the genetic determination of familial diseases and the genetic predisposition of sporadic cases have made enormous advances (for review see Feldman and Gracon[48] and

Mullan and Crawford[66]). Genetic link studies had already shown the genetic heterogeneity of many familial diseases and had allowed the identification of chromosomes 21 and 14 (early cases) and 19 (late cases). In 1991, Hardy demonstrated a mutation on the APP gene located on chromosome 21 and hypothesized that it was the primary cause of the cascade of lesions in two familial cases.[67] Other mutations have been observed in about 20 families around the world.

In 1993, the group led by Allan Roses made a fundamental advance by showing excessive representation of the epsilon 4 allele of apolipoprotein E (ApoE4) in patients with late familial or sporadic AD. This cholesterol-carrying protein plays an important trophic role at the level of the brain, and the gene coding for its production is located on chromosome 19 in the form of three main alleles, epsilon 2, 3 and 4.[68] Furthermore, this protein shows a high affinity for the amyloid protein.[69]

The presence of ApoE4, especially in its homozygotic form (epsilon 4-epsilon 4), increases the risk of AD and probably plays a role in the age of onset and the rate of progression of the disease. Its role in the pathogenesis of SPs and neurofibrillary tangle (NFT) formation, if confirmed, could lead to new therapeutic advances.[70,71] If the effects of ApoE4 on the promotion and neurotoxicity of the A4 amyloid protein and destabilization of microtubules are confirmed, one might conceive of molecules able to reproduce or potentiate the action of ApoE3 in patients who carry the E4 allele. One study has shown that the ApoE4 genotype is associated with a lower probability of cognitive improvement following therapy with tacrine.[72]

Finally, the recent characterization of gene PS-1 (or S-182) on chromosome 14 (early AD)[73] and of gene PS-2 (or STM2) on chromosome 1 (AD of varying age of onset; one of the families was Volga German)[74] marks the entry of AD genetics into the area of presenilins which might play a major role in intracellular 'traffic' of APP. Major advances may derive from this approach.

Oestrogens

The favourable effects of oestrogen therapy on cognitive functions, and the prevention of AD and its treatment, represent a new area of investigation.[75] This hypothesis is based on the beneficial effects of this therapy on memory functions and other cognitive skills of postmenopausal or aged women,[76-78] the increased risk of AD in women with oestrogen deficiencies,[79] and the increased response to cholinergic treatment of women receiving replacement oestrogen treatment.[80] Large therapeutic trials are currently under way to verify this hypothesis. Recent results show that estrogens may regulate APP metabolism favouring non-amyloidogenic pathways[81] and preventing the action of free radicals.[75] A reduced risk of AD for women having reported use of oestrogens has been recently reported in the Baltimore Longitudinal Study of Aging.[82]

Anti-radical therapies

It is generally recognized that the brain is particularly vulnerable to oxidative stress. Recent research suggests an important role of free radicals in the development of the toxicity of the amyloid protein[83] the formation of NFT and eventually neuronal death. The ties between trisomy 21 characterized by an excess of the gene for superoxide dismutase 1 (SOD1) and AD are in keeping with this hypothesis.[84] Oxidative stress may play a role in all stages of the disease; hence the idea of a possible protective role of antioxidant agents.[85] In a more recent trial,[86] a total of 341 patients received the selective monoamine oxidase inhibitor selegiline, alpha-tocopherol, both selegiline and alpha-tocopherol or placebo for 2 years. There were significant delays in the time to the primary outcome (defined as time to the occurrence of death, institutionalization, loss of the ability to perform basic activities of daily living (ADL), or severe dementia) for the patients treated with selegiline, alpha-tocopherol or combination therapy, as compared with the placebo group.

Conclusions

Recent years have witnessed the appearance of many pharmacological agents with definite or probable actions on a disease which until recently was considered totally beyond therapeutic reach. Following the symptomatic agents already available, one can foresee the development of more aetiologically oriented drugs. Physiopathological and genetic approaches are not mutually exclusive and could indeed be complementary. Preventive or early treatment in subjects with measurably high levels of risk factors could be with us in the relatively near future.

References

1. Nouchi F. La maladie d'Alzheimer, nouvelle peur des Françaises. Le Monde 1994; 30 September: p 12.

2. Dartigues JF, Gagnon M, Michel P, et al. Le programme de recherche PAQUID sur l'épidémiologie de la démence. Méthodes et résultats initiaux. Rev Neurol 1991;147:225-30.

3. Letenneur L, Dequae L, Jacqmin H, et al. Prévalence de la démence en Gironde (France). Rev Epidémiol Santè Publique 1993;41:139-45.

4. Prince M. The number of people with dementia is rising quickly. World Alzheimer's Day Bulletin 1997; 21 September.

5. Bachman DL, Wolf PA, Linn R, et al. Prevalence of dementia and probable senile dementia of the Alzheimer's type in the Framingham Study. Neurology 1992;42:115-19.

6. Gauthier S, Montplaisir J, Petit D, et al. Outcome variables in presymptomatic individuals at higher risk of developing Alzheimer disease. Alzheimer Dis Assoc Disord 1996;10(suppl 1):19-21.

7. Rocca WA, Hofman A, Brayne C, et al. Frequency and distribution of Alzheimer's disease in Europe: a collaboration study of 1980-1990 prevalence findings. Ann Neurol 1991;30:381-9.

8. Aisen P, Davis K. The search for disease-modifying treatment for Alzheimer's disease. Neurology 1997;48:S35-41.

9. Bowen FP, Kamienny RS, Burns MM, Yahr MD. Effects of levodopa treatment on concept formation. Neurology 1975;25:701-4.

10. Davies P, Maloney A. Selective loss of central cholinergic neurons in Alzheimer's disease. Lancet 1976:1403.

11. Perry E, Tomlinson BE, Blessed G, Bergmann K, Gibson P, Perry R. Correlation of cholinergic abnormalities with senile plaques and mental test scores in senile dementia. Br Med J 1978;2:1457-9.

12. Terry R, Peck A, DeTeresa R, Schechter R, Houroupian D. Some morphometric aspects of the brain in senile dementia of the Alzheimer type. Ann Neurol 1981;10:184-92.

13. Whitehouse PJ, Price DL, Clark AW, Coyle JT, DeLong MR. Alzheimer's disease: evidence for selective loss of cholinergic neurons in the nucleus basalis. Ann Neurol 1981;10:122-6.

14. Mesulam M, Mufson E, Levey A, Wainer B. Cholinergic innervation of cortex by the basal forebrain. J Comp Neurol 1983;214:170-97.

15. Alzheimer A. Uber Eine eigenartige Erkrankung der Hirnrinde. In: Rottenberg DA, Hochberg FH (eds.) Neurological classics in modern translation. New-York: Hafner Press, 1977:41-3.

16. Gauss CJ. Geburten im Kunstltichem Dammerschlaf. Arch Gynacol 1906:579-93.

17. Drachman D, Leavitt J. Human memory and the cholinergic system: a relationship to aging? Arch Neurol 1974;30:113-21.

18. Signoret J, Whiteley A, Lhermitte F. Influence of choline on amnesia in early Alzheimer's disease. Lancet 1978;2:837.

19. Wurtman RJ, Blusztajn JK, Maire J-C. Autocannibalism' of choline-containing phospholipids in the pathogenesis of Alzheimer's disease; a hypothesis. Neurochem Int 1985;7:369-72.

20. Becker R, Giacobini E, Elbe R, McIlhany M, Sherman K. Potential pharmacotherapy of Alzheimer's disease. A comparison of various forms of physostigamine administration. Acta Neurol Scand 1988;77:19-32.

21. Peterson C, Gibson G. Amelioration of age-related neurochemical and behavioral deficits by 3-4 diaminopyridine. Neurobiol Aging 1983;41:25-43.

22. Tariot PN, Cohen RM, Welkowitz JA, et al. Multiple-dose arecoline infusions in Alzheimer's disease. Arch Gen Psychiatry 1988;45:901-11.

23. Harbaugh R, Roberts D, Coombs DW, Sanders RL, Reeder T. Preliminary report: intracranial cholinergic drug infusion in patients with Alzheimer's disease. Neurosurgery 1984;15:514-18.

24. Penn R, Martin E, Wilson R, Fox JH, Savoy S. Intraventricular bethanecol infusion for Alzheimer' disease. Results of double-blind and escalating-dose trial. Neurology 1988;38:219-22.

25. Sahakian J, Levy R. The effect of nicotine on attention, information processing and short term memory in patients with dementia of the Alzheimer type. Br J Psychiatry 1989;154:797-800.

26. Court J, Perry E. Dementia: the neurochemical basis of putative transmitter orientated therapy. Pharmcol Ther 1991;52:423-43.

27. Smith C, Swash M. Hypothesis—possible biochemical basis of memory disorders in Alzheimer's disease. Ann Neurol 1978;3:471-3.

28. Becker R, Giacobini E, Elble R, McIlhany M, Sherman K. Potential pharmacotherapy of Alzheimer disease. A comparison of various forms of physostigmine administration. Acta Neurol Scand 1988;77:19-32.

29. Beller S, Overall J, Rhodes H, Swann A. Long-term outpatient treatment of senile dementia with physostigmine. J Clin Psychiatry 1988;49:400-4.

30. Thal L, Fuld P, Masur M, Sharples N. Oral physostigmine and lecithin improve memory in Alzheimer's disease. Ann Neurol 1983;13:491-6.

31. Albert A, Rubbo S, Goldacre R, Davey M, Stone J. The influence of chemical constitution on antibacterial activity. Part II: A general survey of the acridine series. Br J Exp Pathol 1945;26:160-92.

32. Thornton J, Gershon S. The history of THA. In: Giacobini E, Becker R, eds. Current research in Alzheimer therapy. New York: Taylor and Francis, 1988: 267-78.

33. Drukarch B, Kits K, Van der Meer E, et al. 9-Amino 1,2,3,4-tetrahydroxyacridine (THA), an alleged drug for the treatment of Alzheimer's disease, inhibits acetylcholinesterase activity and slow outward K$^+$ current. Eur J Pharmacol 1987;141:153-7.

34. Bowen D, Steele J, Lowe S, Palmer A. Tacrine in relation to aminoacid transmitters in Alzheimer's disease. In: Wurtman R, Corkin S, Growdon J, Ritter-Walker E, eds. Fifth meeting of the International Study Group on the Pharmacology of Memory

Disorders associated with aging. (Zurich, 1989):147-57.

35. Kaye W, Sitaram N, Weingartner H, Ebert M, Smallberg S, Gillin J. Modest facilitation of memory in dementia with combined lecithin and anticholinesterase treatment. Biol Psychiatry 1982;17:275-80.

36. Summers W, Viesselman J, Marsh G, Candelora K. Use of THA in treatment of Alzheimer-like dementia: pilot study in twelve patients. Biol Psychiatry 1981;16:145-53.

37. Summers W, Majovski V, Marsh G, Tachiki K, Kling A. Oral tetrahydroaminoacridine in long-term treatment of senile dementia. N Engl J Med 1986;315:1241-5.

38. Davis KL, Thal LJ, Gamzu ER, et al. A double-blind, placebo-controlled multicenter study of tacrine for Alzheimer's disease. N Engl J Med 1992;327:1253-9.

39. Forette F, Hoover T, Gracon S, et al. A double-blind, placebo-controlled, enriched population study of tacrine in patients with Alzheimer's disease. Eur J Neurol 1995;2:229-38.

40. Knapp MJ, Knopman DS, Solomon PR, Pendlebury WW, Davis CS, Gracon SI. A 30-week randomized controlled trial of high-dose tacrine in patients with Alzheimer's disease. JAMA 1994;271:985-91.

41. Knopman D, Schneider L, Davis K, et al. Long-term tacrine (Cognex TM) treatment effects on nursing home placement and mortality. Neurology 1996;47:166-77.

42. Giacobini E, Zhu XD, Williams E, Ka S. The effect of the selective reversible acetylcholinesterase inhibitor E2020 on extracellular acetylcholine and biogenic amine levels in rat cortex. Neuropharmacology 1996;35:205-11.

43. Rogers S, Farlow M, Doody RS, et al. A 24 week double-blind placebo-controlled trial of donepezil in patients with Alzheimer's disease. Neurology 1998;50:136-45.

44. Anand R, Gharabawi G. Efficacy and safety results of the early phase studies with Exelon (ENA 713) in Alzheimer's disease: an overview. J Drug Dev Clin Pract 1996;8:1-14.

45. Bassant M, Jazat-Poindessous F, Lamour Y. Effects of metrifonate, a cholinesterase inhibitor, on local cerebral glucose utilization in young and aged rats. J Cereb Blood Flow Metab 1996;16:1014-25.

46. Becker R, Colliver J, Markwell S, Moriearty P, Unni L, Vicari S. Double-blind, placebo-controlled study of metrifonate, an acetylcholinesterase inhibitor, for Alzheimer disease. Alzheimer Dis Assoc Disord 1996;10:124-31.

47. Tariot P, Schneider L. Clinical reviews: Contemporary treatment approaches to Alzheimer's disease. Consult Pharm 1996;11(suppl E):16-24.

48. Feldman H, Gracon S. Alzheimer's disease: symptomatic drugs under development. In: Gauthier S, ed. Clinical diagnosis and management of Alzheimer's disease. London: Martin Dunitz Ltd, 1996:239-59.

49. Coull JT. Pharmacological manipulations of the alpha2 noradrenergic system. Effect on cognition. Drugs Aging 1994;5:116-26.

50. Bissette G, Myers B. Minireview. Somatostatin in Alzheimer's disease and depression. Life Sci 1992;51:1389-410.

51. Izquierdo I. Role of NMDA receptors in memory. Trends Pharmacol Sci 1991;12:128-9.

52. Boller F, Forette F, Khatchaturian Z, Poncet M, Christen Y. Heterogeneity of Alzheimer's disease. Berlin Heidelberg, New York: Springer Verlag, 1992.

53. Shvaloff A, Neuman E, Guez D. Lines of therapeutics research in Alzheimer's disease. Psychopharmacol Bull 1996;32:343-52.

54. McGeer P, McGeer E. The inflammatory response system of the brain: implications for therapy of Alzheimer and other neurodegenerative disease. Brain Res Rev 1995;21:195-218.

55. Breitner JCS, Gau MSW, Welsh KA, et al. Inverse association of anti-inflammatory treatments and Alzheimer's disease, Neurology 1994;44:227-32.

56. Rich JB, Rasmusson DX, Folstein MF, Carson KA, Kawas C, Brandt J. Nonsteroidal anti-inflammatory drugs in Alzheimer's disease. Neurology 1995;45:51-5.

57. Rogers J, Kirby LC, Hempelman SR, et al. Clinical trial of indomethacin in Alzheimer's disease. Neurology 1993;43:1609-11.

58. Tollefson GD. Short term effect of the calcium blocker nimodipine in the management of primary degenerative dementia. Biol. Psychiatry 1990;27:1133-42.

59. Olson L. Growth factors: therapeutic implications. In: Forette FCY, Boller F, eds. Cerebral Plasticity and Cognitive Stimulation (Fondation Nationale de Gérontologie: Paris, 1993) 32-44.

60. Hefti IR, Schneider LS. Rationale for the planned clinical trials with nerve growth factor in Alzheimer's disease. Psychiatr Dev 1989;4:299-315.

61. Winkler J, Thal L. Clinical potential of growth factors in neurological disorders. CNS Drugs 1994;6:465-78.

62. Yankner BA, Duffy LK, Kirshner DA. Neurotrophic and neurotoxic effects of amyloid beta protein: reversal by tachykinin neuropeptides. Science 1990;250:279-82.

63. Hardy J, Allsop D. Amyloid deposition as the central event in the aetiology of Alzheimer's disease. Trends Pharmacol Sci 1991;12:383-8.

64. Allain H, Belliard S, de Certaines J, Bentué-Ferrer D, Bureau M, Lacroix P. Potential biological targets for anti-Alzheimer drugs. Dementia 1993;4:347-52.

65. Maury CPJ. Biology of disease. Molecular pathogenesis of beta-amyloidosis in Alzheimer's disease and other cerebral amyloidosis. Lab Invest 1995;72:4-16.

66. Mullan M, Crawford F. The molecular genetics of Alzheimer's disease. Mol Biol 1994;9:15-22.

67. Chartier-Harlin M, Crawford F, Houlden H, et al. Early onset Alzheimer's disease caused by mutation at codon 717 of the beta amyloid precursor protein gene. Nature 1991;353:844-6.

68. Saunders AM, Strittmatter WJ, Schmechel DE, et al. Association of apolipoprotein E allele $\epsilon4$ with late-onset familial and sporadic Alzheimer's disease. Neurology 1993;43:1467-72.

69. Strittmatter WJ, Saunders AM, Schmechel DE, Pericak-Vance MA, Roses AD. Apolipoprotein E: high

affinity binding to βA amyloid and increased frequency of type 4 allele in familial Alzheimer's disease. Proc Natl Acad Sci USA 1993;90:1977-81.

70. Hardy J. Apoliprotein E in the genetics and epidemiology of Alzheimer's disease. Am J Med Genet 1995;60:456-60.

71. Roses A. Perspective. On the metabolism of apolipoprotein E and the Alzheimer diease. Exp Neurol 1995;132:149-56.

72. Farlow M, Lahiri D, Poirier J, Davignon J, Hui S. Apolipoprotein E genotype and gender influence response to tacrine therapy. Ann NY Acad Sci 1996;802:101-10.

73. Sherrington R, Rogaev EI, Liang Y, et al. Cloning of a gene bearing missense mutations in early onset familial Alzheimer's disease. Nature 1995;375:754-60.

74. Levy-Lahad E, Wasco W, Poorkaj P, et al. Candidate gene for the chromosome 1 familial Alzheimer's disease locus. Science 1995;269:973-7.

75. Fillit H. Future therapeutic developments of estrogene use. J Clin Pharmacol 1995;35:25S-8S.

76. Robinson D, Fireadman L, Marcus R. Estrogen replacement therapy and memory in older women. J Am Geriatr Soc 1994;42:919-22.

77. Henderson W, Paganini-Hill A, Emanuel CK, Dunn ME, Galen Buckwalter J. Estrogen replacement therapy in older women. Comparisons between Alzheimer's disease cases and nondemented control subjects. Arch Neurol 1994;51:896-900.

78. Henderson V, Watt L, Buckwalter J. Cognitive skills associated with estrogen replacement in women with Alzheimer's disease. Psychoneuroendocrinology 1996;21:421-30.

79. Paganini-Hill A, Henderson W. Estrogen deficiency and risk of Alzheimer's disease. Am J Epidemiol 1994;140:256-61.

80. Schneider L, Farlow MR. Predicting response to cholinesterase inhibitors. Possible approaches. CNS Drugs 1995;4:114-24.

81. Jaffe AB, Toran-Allerand D, Greengard P. Estrogen regulates metabolism of Alzheimer amyloid beta precursor protein. J Biol Chem 1994;269:13065-8.

82. Kawas C, Resnick S, Morrison A, et al. A prospective study of estrogen replacement therapy and the risk of developing Alzheimer's disease. Neurology 1997;48:1517-21.

83. Iversen LL, Mortishire-Smith RJ, Pollack SJ. The toxicity in vitro of beta amyloid protein. Biochem J 1995;311:1-16.

84. Sinet PM, Ceballos-Picot I. Role of free radicals in Alzheimer's disease and Down's syndrome. In: Packer L, Prilikpo L, Christen Y, eds. Free radicals in the brain (Berlin, Heidelberg, New York: Springer Verlag, 1992) 91-8.

85. Kagan VE, Bakalova RA, Koynova GM. Antioxidant protection of the brain against oxidative stress. In: Packer L, Prilikpo L, Christen Y, eds. Free radicals in the brain (Berlin, Heidelberg, New York: Springer Verlag, 1992) 49-61.

86. Sano M, Ernesto C, Thomas R, et al. A controlled trial of selegiline, alpha-tocopherol, or both as treatment for Alzheimer's disease. The Alzheimer's Disease Cooperative Study. N Engl J Med 1997;336:1216-22.

The natural progression of Alzheimer's disease

Carolina Piccini, Laura Bracco and Luigi Amaducci

Introduction

The notion that, on the clinical level, Alzheimer's disease (AD) corresponds mainly to an aphasic–apraxic–agnosic syndrome is no longer deemed tenable; rather, the conviction is growing that we are dealing with a heterogeneous disorder in terms of clinical pattern, disease progression and, probably, response to therapy.

The development of well-defined standarized sets of criteria[1-3] and their wide adoption have made the clinical diagnosis of AD more stringent.[4] Furthermore, since the greater emphasis on early diagnosis, patients are now followed up from the beginning of their symptoms until the terminal stages of the disease. The relatively disappointing results of previous clinical trials devoted to the improvement of cognitive functions in AD suggested that an arrest or slowing of progressive deterioration could be a more feasible aim of a biological treatment.[5] Therefore, data arising from clinical and epidemiological research on AD represent, in planning clinical trials, the indispensable background of knowledge to guide an accurate selection of cases and appropriate instruments to evaluate the efficacy of treatments. This can only be assessed by having more precise information about the variability of the clinical course of the disease and by knowing its natural progression in the absence of specific interventions. On this basis, research has been focused on the necessity of longitudinal studies in order to allow a detailed description of patients' cognitive deficits and progression of functional decline.

The clinical course of Alzheimer's disease

The typical course of AD is characterized by the impairment of memory and other cognitive functions—language, orientation, constructional abilities, abstract thinking, problem-solving and praxis—that must be of sufficient severity to interfere with occupational and/or social performance and that may be associated with behavioural disturbances (DSM-IV). An insidious onset of symptoms with a progressive decline has been regarded as the

hallmark of AD, as compared to vascular dementia.

Cross-sectional studies, looking at patients with different degrees of dementia severity, provided the basis for a model of progression through different stages of the disease characterized by certain clusters of cognitive and functional symptoms. Although such a model has been largely adopted as representing the typical course of AD, it is now clear that frequent deviations from the classical progression occur. Furthermore, we should bear in mind that an early identification of cognitive impairments depends in large part on the experience of the physician and on the availability of psychometric instruments of sufficient sensitivity for unequivocal deficits to emerge. For instance, deficits in attention, judgement and problem-solving, although present from the beginning of the disease, are too complex to be assessed clinically and have only recently been investigated more systematically, since the involvement of the frontal lobe has been considered to be part of AD.

The memory deficit, first complained of subjectively and then objectively demonstrated, is the early and pivotal symptom of AD, with a poor performance especially on tests of delayed recall of verbal memory—the most sensitive tests to distinguish early AD from normal controls.[6-8] In a variable percentage of cases it may be associated with depression of mood which gives rise to the problem of differential diagnosis. Four possibilities have been considered in order to explain the relationship between dementia and depression: depression could be a psychological reaction of patients to the awareness of their own deficits; depression and cognitive deficits may be different symptoms of a single disease or an incidental association of two diseases; or, finally, memory complaints as well as the poor performance on memory tests may result from the mood disorder itself, i.e. 'pseudodementia'.[9] All of these hypotheses could be true in different patients, with different implications for disease progression: while in the first case loss of insight should improve the affective disorder despite the progression of cognitive decline, in the case of pseudodementia the cognitive impairment should reverse in response to antidepressant therapy. Furthermore, the psychological reaction of the early stages could be replaced in the later stages by a mood disorder that is now regarded as a behavioural disturbance.

The progressive involvement of different cognitive domains, as described by clinical and neuropsychological observations, is supported by the notion, arising from pathological and morphofunctional studies,[10-12] of an early involvement of the mesial temporal lobes followed by the disruption of temporoparietal and frontal association cortices with a relative preservation of the primary motor cortex.

Although great emphasis has been placed on a hierarchical progression of symptoms in the typical course of AD (Table 2.1), it is now clear that different cognitive and non-cognitive domains may be affected in each patient, with different timing of onset and progression. The emergence of atypical clinical profiles has been largely investigated in relation to prognosis and rate of disease progression (see below).

Along with cognitive decline, functional decline, which refers to the progressive loss of ability to perform activities of daily living (ADL), is a significant feature of AD. This loss of functional abilities in hierarchical—complex instrumental activities (such as dealing with finances) are lost before the basic ADL. Progressive losses in basic ADL generally correspond to moderate and severe

Table 2.1
Hierarchical progression of symptoms in AD.

Early stages
 Minimal temporal disorientation
 Difficulty in recalling recent events
 Word-finding difficulty in spontaneous speech with relative sparing of comprehension
 Constructional apraxia for tridimensional drawings
 Anxiety/denial/depression
 Difficulty at work
 No motor disturbances

Intermediate stages
 Temporospatial disorientation
 Moderate–severe memory deficit interfering with activities of daily living (i.e. shopping)
 Increasing language impairment (paraphasias, anomia, circumlocutions,
  comprehension deficits)
 Constructional apraxia
 Ideational/ideomotor apraxia, dressing apraxia
 Agnosia
 Behavioural disturbances (delusions, hallucinations, paranoid symptoms, wandering)
 Bradykinesia, extrapyramidal signs
 Decreased interest in toileting

Late stages
 Cognitive abilities are completely lost, with difficulty in recognizing familiar faces or
  spaces
 Language range from a semantic jargon to a complete mutism
 Rigidity, bradykinesia, seizure, myoclonus
 Aggressive behaviour, wandering, hallucinations
 Total dependency in toileting, dressing and feeding
 Sphincteric incontinence

degrees of cognitive impairment as described by Reisberg in the Global Deterioration Scale and in the Functional Assessment Staging.[13,14] The ability to dress, bath and toilet decreases progressively, with a generally belated loss of feeding ability; in the latest stages, sphincteric incontinence appears with sequential loss of basic motor capacity (such as ability to stand or sit up, to smile and to hold up the head). Assessment of functional abilities, mainly investigated by means of informant-based instruments, is important for dementia diagnosis and may help the staging of dementia severity, since functional abilities decline over a period of several years. Furthermore, since the declines in cognitive and functional abilities are not necessarily parallel, independent evaluations of these two aspects should be carried out in a comprehensive assessment of disease progression.

Behavioural alterations such as hallucinations, delusional jealousy, screaming, agitation, aggressive behaviour, misidentification and depression, already studied as possible prognostic factors or markers of AD subgroups,[15] are now investigated more systematically because they represent a major source of caregiver burden and failure of home care. These symptoms, first described in the original report by Alois Alzheimer, occur in most patients with AD and have been reported with high variability. This variability is mostly due to bias of research on clinical samples and to difficulties in recording and grouping symptoms.[16] On this basis, comprehensive and sensitive instruments to detect and quantify

neuropsychiatric disturbances have been recently developed.[17] Behavioural alterations, regarded in the past as typical of the advanced stages of the disease only, have been instead observed throughout, from the early to the later stages of the disease, with a spike of occurrence in the moderate phase.[18]

The idea that AD progresses in a hierarchical fashion has largely contributed to and theoretically supported the search of clinical milestones. Researchers have shifted their attention from long-term end-points, such as institutionalization, sphincteric incontinence or death, which have been adopted for survival analysis, to short- and medium-term clinical end-points useful for clinical and therapeutic studies. Precise criteria for the definition of such clinical milestones have been discussed and, in the experience of the Consortium to Establish a Registry for Alzheimer's Disease (CERAD), some clinical features have been investigated to identify those able to chart the progression of AD throughout its course, overcoming problems such as ceiling and floor effects typical of psychometric test scores. Valid end-points should be unambiguous, be clinically relevant, be common and cover the whole course of the disease, and be primarily related to disease progression, with no reversal. Unfortunately, none of the investigated 'clinical events' fulfil completely all of the selected criteria. Nevertheless, decline in Clinical Dementia Rating,[19] loss of instrumental ADL (IADL), failure to recall three words as well as a decline in total score on the Minimum Mental State Examination (MMSE)[20] and a score below 10 on the MMSE were 'high-risk milestones'; IADL and basic ADL are lost in a hierarchical manner, although they are not able to cover the disease course with regular spacing. In conclusion, the authors suggest that clinical milestones could be combined with the evaluation of cognitive change in order to achieve greater accuracy in charting either natural progression of efficacy of treatments.[21]

Disease progression and prognostic factors: the contribution of the longitudinal studies

Research on AD has entered a phase in which high priority is being given to longitudinal studies, which are necessary to investigate appropriately an evolving process.

Disease progression

Among the pivotal issues to be addressed by longitudinal surveys is the definition of disease progression. The rate at which dementia progresses might serve as an additional aid to diagnosis and as a variable to identify AD clinical subtypes. We know that in clinical diagnosis the timing of cognitive decline is extremely important in terms of both onset and progression. The progressive nature of the disease through stages involving mood, cognition, functional autonomy, behaviour and loss of motor skills has been considered one of the most relevant and typical features of AD. Nevertheless, longitudinal observations have shown a variability in the course of the disease.

The issue of progression, first investigated in terms of survival and identification of prognostic factors, was later studied by refinement in the rate of change, calculated as the difference between the initial and final score of a patient on a cognitive or functional scale, divided by the intervening years, and generally expressed as mean points lost per year.

In the last revision of the *Diagnostic and Statistical Manual of Mental Disorders*,[1] the disease progression is characterized as 'a loss of 3–4 points per year on MMSE'. Despite this explicit statement, the definition of a typical rate of change on cognitive and functional scales is rather questionable and is affected by several methodological and theoretical problems. First of all, the definition of the change over time requires follow-up of sufficient duration as well as reliable and valid instruments of measurement. Clinical as well as research data support the notion of an extremely variable patient performance on repeated exposure to psychometric tests such as the MMSE.[22] Therefore, only by knowing the within-subject variability is it possible to interpret correctly the true amount of change.[23] Although instruments such as the MMSE and the Information Memory Concentration Test (IMCT)[24] have been widely applied to measure the rate of change of cognitive decline, more extensive evaluation (i.e. WAIS) resulted in a more reliable measure of the progression.[25] Recent research has focused on the different contribution of several neuropsychological tests in describing disease progression: while tests such as those exploring explicit memory have an early floor effect, as suggested by a decelerating curve-to-floor effect pattern of progression, tests showing linear decline over time are best

for tracking the course of the disease— i.e. the IMCT, Boston Naming Test, Verbal Fluency Test and Boston Visual Retention Test.[8]

The model of progression that has been mostly applied in the study of disease progression is a linear one. Although it has been a good first step to analyse the disease progression, it is based on the implicit assumption that cognitive decline is steadily linear over time. Trilinear as well as curvilinear models have been proposed to better represent the natural course of the disease.[26,27]

The high inter- and intrasubject variability, already demonstrated by clinical studies[28–43] (Table 2.2), has been further supported by neuroimaging longitudinal studies on rate of change of cerebral atrophy. The longitudinal determination of ventricular volume[44] as well as the rate of change of cerebral atrophy on brain CT or MR scans[45,46] have been recently considered not only for the potential advantage of increased diagnostic specificity, but also as a measure of disease progression in clinical trials.

Finally, there must be cautious application of data derived from clinical trials. For instance, the cognitive subscale of the Alzheimer's Disease Assessment

Table 2.2
Annual rate of change for cognitive and functional scales.

Reference no.	Sample size	Study length (years)	MMSE (points/ year)	IMCT (points/ year)	BDS (points/ year)
28	40	5	–	4.5 (3.1)	–
29[a]	161	2	–	4.4 (3.6)	–
31	30	–	4.2[b]	–	–
30	44	1	1.8[b]	–	–
32[a]	54	1	–	4.1 (3.0)	–
35[a]	106	1	2.8 (4.6)	–	–
34[a]	92	2	2.8 (4.3)	3.2 (3.0)	–
33	53	–	–	–	1.5[b]
36[a]	65	4	4.5[b]	–	–
37	110	1	3.5 (5.9)	2.8	–
38[a]	111	8	–	4.1[b]	–
39[a]	44	–	1.8[b]	–	–
40	90	1	4.3[b]	–	–
41	56	1	–	2.6 (4.9)	3.5 (3.7)
42	104	–	–	5.3 (5.0)	–
43	31	7	–	4.4 (3.2)	–

[a] These studies take into consideration that fact that the rate of change varies with disease severity.
[b] Standard deviations not available.
BDS, Blessed Dementia Scale; IMCT, Information Memory Concentration Test; MMSE, Mini Mental State Examination.
Values are mean annual rate of change in test performance (points/year); standard deviations are in parentheses.

Scale (ADAS)[47] has become the standard instrument for demonstrating cognitive improvement in short-term efficacy AD drug trials since it was used for the approval of tacrine in 1992 and of donepezil in 1997. Although the double-blind design of a clinical trial allows a direct comparison with the placebo group, few data have been acquired on the effects of various demographic or clinical variables on ADAS-Cog perfor-mance[48,49] and on the natural decline of performance on this scale. Data arising from analysis of patients in the placebo arm should be cautiously adopted to describe such a decline, since it may be affected by the participation in a clinical trial per se.[50]

Prognostic factors

Several longitudinal studies have sought to identify predictors of death as well as of cognitive and functional decline in patients with AD and to evaluate the prognostic value of certain clinical features. Demographic characteristics such as age, gender and education have been investigated.

Early age of onset has been positively correlated with a rapid progression and shorter survival,[51-54] although the opposite relation has also been reported[55] and several authors found no effect of age on the course of the disease.[29,37,56] In the CERAD experience, from a large data set the role of age of onset has been further investigated in terms of differences in clinical and neuropsychological features: when age is treated as a continuous variable, and severity of dementia is controlled for, a younger age of onset has been reported to be significantly related to a poor performance on measures of language and concentration on entry into the study and to be a predictor of a significantly faster rate of progression.[54]

As far as gender is concerned, although males affected by AD have a shorter survival than non-demented controls, it does not appear to imply differences in disease progression.[29,37,53,57] Nevertheless, recent studies have reported a possible interaction between gender and apolipoprotein E (ApoE) genotype, which is known to affect age of onset—younger in ApoE4-positive women[58]—as well as the response to pharmacological treatment.[59] Furthermore, another factor that could modify the natural course of the disease and the response to pharmacological treatment in females is exposure to oestrogen replacement therapy, which appears to prevent or delay onset of dementia[60-62] and to enhance the response to cholinesterase inhibitors[63]—see Birge for an extensive review.[64]

While lack of education has been reported as a major risk factor for and determinant of prevalence of dementia in some studies,[65-67] the possible role of education in AD and, in particular, in AD progression remains uncertain.[29,36,53,57,68-71]

Among clinical features, extrapyramidal signs (EPS)—mainly bradykinesia and rigidity—as well as psychotic symptoms have been well investigated[15,38,53,72,73] and have been reported in an increasing amount of cases (20–50%), especially since longitudinal surveys have allowed the detection of their development in the later stages of the disease.[53,73] There is controversy concerning whether EPS and psychosis are predictors of a faster decline or are simply signs in the course of the disease representing a stage-dependent manifestation of AD. The application of statistical analysis able to control for dementia severity has led to the suggestion that EPS and psychosis are predictors of a more rapid course of AD, although some studies did not confirm this finding.[37,57] Nevertheless, the presence of EPS could mark the presence of a second neurodegenerative disorder or may represent a distinct pathological subtype, the so-called Lewy body variant. Although EPS have sometimes been associated with pathological changes in the brainstem, including AD pathology, Lewy bodies, or neuronal loss in the substantia nigra, their pathological basis remains uncertain. An early appearance of spontaneous Parkinsonism may suggest a different diagnosis (i.e. dementia of Lewy body type, DLB) or AD with a poorer prognosis. The faster progression and the good response to tacrine of DLB make imperative an accurate diagnosis of such cases by means of the recently revised diagnostic criteria.[74]

Neuropsychological characterization of AD patients has been a matter of great interest, and different patterns of cognitive impairment have been considered in order to identify neuropsychological subtyes and to evaluate their potential value in predicting the course of the disease. Some studies have reported a faster decline for patients with a predominant impairment of language ability,[30,36,57] while others have suggested a poorer prognosis for those cases with severe visuospatial disorders.[37,54] When patients are selected on the basis of the rate of progression of mental decline, 'faster decliners' have been reported to display a greater impairment of executive functions and a significant reduction of frontal metabolism in comparison to 'slower decliners'.[75] Research in this field has focused attention on the existence of various subgroups of individuals who, initially and/or consistently over time, present specific patterns of deficits. In particular, cases with focal deficit and relative sparing of other cognitive functions have been identified (i.e. temporal lobe dysfunction, semantic dementia). The observed differences in rate of decline of these cases—although it remains unclear whether they represent a clinical or a biological variant—emphasize the relevance of a detailed and comprehensive neuropsychological assessment in selecting cases for clinical pharmacological trials.[76]

The search for prognostic factors and for clinical subgroups/subtypes has brought to light the problem of whether the observed differences were the result of different degrees of disease severity or of a true subtyping.[38,77,78] Several studies have reported that the initial degree of severity (how far) rather than the historical rate of progression (how fast) best predicts the time to reach clinical endpoints.[21,56,57,79] Nevertheless, other studies indicate that the rate of progression of cognitive decline appears to be as strong a predictor of the clinical course of the disease as initial disease severity.[80]

Among possible biological markers of AD investigated in the recent years the ApoE genotype now appears to be the most relevant, and is a major source of controversy among clinicians and researchers.[81]

Since 1994, many studies have reported an association between the ApoE4 allele and an increased risk of developing sporadic and familial late-onset AD as well as a possible protective effect of the ApoE2 allele—see Farlow for an update.[82] The frequency of the ApoE4 genotype in AD cases is three times that in non-demented age-matched controls, and the age of onset of AD appears to decrease with increasing ApoE4 gene dose. Furthermore, the ApoE4 allele has been reported to influence the natural course of AD, although with controversial results. Studies on patients with an isolated memory deficit[83] or minimal cognitive impairment[84] have reported a higher rate of developing probable AD in ApoE4 carriers. Other studies, focused on rate of change of cognitive decline in AD cases, failed to confirm any influence of the ApoE4 genotype status on rate of progression of mental decline,[85,86] while others report an inverse relationship[87] (homozygous ApoE4/4 cases progress with only 2.2 points lost per year on the MMSE, in comparison with 3.8 and 4.7 points per year lost by heterozygous ApoE4 and non-ApoE4 AD cases).[88] Such data, as well as those that suggest that ApoE2 and ApoE3 AD cases could respond better to cholinesterase therapy,[59] call for further studies on this issue and underline the need to consider the ApoE genotype in the design of clinical trials.

Among neuroimaging features investigated for their potential role in determining the clinical pattern of the prognosis of AD, frontal hypometabolism[75] as well as temporal hypometabolism[89] have been reported to be related to a faster progression, while white matter changes and silent strokes show no clear relation with the progression of the disease.[90,91]

Conclusions

The increasing number of new treatments of AD requires careful re-examination of clinical trial designs. Given the rather modest results in symptomatic therapy for AD patients, a main objective of treatment could be to slow the progression of cognitive and functional decline. The assessment of the course of the disease thus becomes essential. The convergence of different lines of evidence—genetic, clinical, morphological, functional—is now bringing into even sharper focus the heterogeneity of AD. New data on rate of progression have revealed a high intra- and intersubject variability, underlining the need for an accurate selection of sensitive measures of change.[92] Furthermore, difficulties in cognitive change quantification suggest the opportunity of evaluating aspects other than cognitive decline, such as ADL, behaviour or caregivers' time use.[93] Thus, patterns of clinical presentation, rates of progression and prognostic factors should be considered in the design and analysis of clinical trials.

References

1. Diagnostic and Statistical Manual of Mental Disorders, 4th edn (The American Psychiatric Association: Washington DC, 1994).

2. International Statistical Classification of Diseases, 10th revision ICD-10 (World Health Organization: Geneva, 1992).

3. McKhann G, Drachman D, Folstein M, Katzman R, Price D, Stadlan EM. Clinical diagnosis of Alzheimer's disease: report of the NINCDS–ADRDA Work Group under the auspices of the Department of Health and Human Services Task Force on Alzheimer's Disease. Neurology 1984;34:939–44.

4. Gearing M, Mirra SS, Hedreen JC, Sumi SM, Hansen LA, Heyman A. The Consortium to Establish a Registry of Alzheimer's Disease (CERAD). Part X. Neuropathology confirmation of the clinical diagnosis of Alzheimer's disease. Neurology 1995;45:461–6.

5. Swash M, Brooks DN, Day NE, Frith CD, Levy R, Warlow CP. Clinical trials in Alzheimer's disease. A report from the MRC Alzheimer's Disease Clinical Trials Committee. J Neurol Neurosurg Psychiatry 1991;54:178–81.

6. Bracco L, Amaducci L, Pedone D, et al. Italian Multicentre Study on Dementia (SMID): a neuropsychological test battery for assessing Alzheimer's disease. J Psychiatr Res 1990;24:213–26.

7. Welsh KA, Butters N, Hughes JP, Mohs RC, Heyman A. Detection and staging of dementia in Alzheimer's disease: use of the neuropsychological measures developed for the Consortium to Establish a Registry for Alzheimer's disease. Arch Neurol 1992;49:448-52.

8. Locascio JJ, Growdon JH, Corkin S. Cognitive test performance in detecting, staging and tracking Alzheimer's disease. Arch Neurol 1995;52:1087-99.

9. Kramer SI, Reifler BV. Depression, dementia and reversible dementia. Clin Geriatr Med 1992;8:289-97.

10. Braak H, Braak E. Evolution of the neuropathology of Alzheimer's disease. Acta Neurol Scand Suppl 1996;165:3-12.

11. Haxby JV, Grady CL, Friedland RP, Rapoport SI. Neocortical metabolic abnormalities precede non memory cognitive impairments in early dementia of the Alzheimer type: longitudinal confirmation. J Neural Transm 1987;24(suppl):49-53.

12. Jagust WJ. Functional imaging in dementia: an overview. J Clin Psychiatry 1994;55(suppl):5-11.

13. Reisberg B, Ferris SH, deLeon MJ, Crook T. Global Deterioration Scale (GDS). Psychopharmacol Bull 1988;24:661-3.

14. Reisberg B. Functional assessment staging (FAST). Psychopharmacol Bull 1988;24:653-9.

15. Mayeux R, Stern Y, Spanton S. Heterogeneity in dementia of the Alzheimer's type: evidence of subgroups. Neurology 1985;35:453-61.

16. Borson S, Raskind MA. Clinical features and pharmacologic treatment of behavioural symptoms of Alzheimer's disease. Neurology 1997;48(suppl):S17-24.

17. Cummings JL. The neuropsychiatric inventory: assessing psychopathology in dementia patients. Neurology 1997;48(suppl 6):S10-16.

18. Mega MS, Cummings JL, Fiorello T, Gorbein J. The spectrum of behavioural changes in Alzheimer's disease. Neurology 1996;46:130-5.

19. Morris JC. The Clinical Dementia Rating (CDR): current version and scoring rules. Neurology 1993;43:2412-14.

20. Folstein MF, Folstein SE, McHugh PR. 'Mini Mental State': a practical method for grading the cognitive state of patients for the clinicians. J Psychiatr Res 1975;12:189-98.

21. Galasko D, Edland SD, Morris JC, Clark C, Mohs R, Koss E. The Consortium to Establish a Registry for Alzheimer's Disease (CERAD): Part XI. Clinical milestones in patients with Alzheimer's disease followed over 3 years. Neurology 1995;45:1451-5.

22. van Belle G, Uhlmann RF, Hughes JP, Larson EB. Reliability of estimates of changes in mental status test performance in senile dementia of the Alzheimer type. J Clin Epidemiol 1990;43:589-95.

23. Knopman D, Gracon S. Observation on the short-term 'natural history' of probable Alzheimer's disease in controlled clinical trials. Neurology 1994;44:260-5.

24. Blessed G, Tomlinson BE, Roth M. The association between quantitative measures of dementia and of senile change in the cerebral grey matter of elderly subjects. Br J Psychiatry 1968;114:797-811.

25. Haxby JV, Raffaele K, Gillette J, Schapiro MB, Rapoport SI. Individual trajectories of cognitive decline in patients with dementia of Alzheimer type. J Clin Exp Neuropsychiatry 1992;14:575-92.

26. Brooks JO, Kraemer HC, Tanke ED, Yesavage JA. The methodology of studying decline in Alzheimer's disease. J Am Geriatr Soc 1993;41:623-8.

27. Helmes E, Merskey H, Fox H, et al. Patterns of deterioration in senile dementia of the Alzheimer type. Arch Neurol 1995;52:306-10.

28. Thal LJ, Grundman M, Klauber MR. Dementia: characteristics of a referral population and factors associated with progression. Neurology 1988;38:1083-90.

29. Katzman R, Brown T, Thal LJ, et al. Comparison of rate of annual change of mental status score in four independent studies of patients with Alzheimer's disease. Ann Neurol 1988;24:384-9.

30. Becker JT, Huff FJ, Nebes RD, Holland A, Boller F. Neuropsychological function in Alzheimer's disease: pattern of impairment and rates of progression. Arch Neurol 1988;45:263-8.

31. Yesavage JA, Poulsen AB, Sheikh J, et al. Rates of change of common measures of impairment in senile dementia of the Alzheimer's type. Psychopharmacol Bull 1988;24:531-4.

32. Ortof E, Crystal HA. Rate of progression of Alzheimer's disease. J Am Geriatr Soc 1989; 37:511-14.

33. Huff FJ, Belle SH, Shim YK, et al. Prevalence and prognostic value of neurologic abnormalities in Alzheimer's disease. Dementia 1990;1:32-40.

34. Salmon DP, Thal LJ, Butters N, Heindel WC. Longitudinal evaluation of dementia of the Alzheimer type: a comparison of 3 standardized mental status examinations. Neurology 1990;40:1225-30.

35. Teri L, Hughes JP, Larson EB. Cognitive deterioration in Alzheimer's disease: behavioral and health factors. J Gerontol 1990;45:58-63.

36. Boller F, Becker JT, Holland AL, Forbes MM, Hood PC, McGonigle-Gibson KL. Predictors of decline in AD. Cortex 1991;27:9-17.

37. Burns A, Jacoby R, Levy R. Progression of cognitive impairment in Alzheimer's disease. J Am Geriatr Soc 1991;39:39.

38. Mortimer JA, Ebbitt B, Jun SJ, Finch MD. Predictors of cognitive and functional progression in patients with probable Alzheimer's disease. Neurology 1992;42:1689-96.

39. Morris JC, Edland S, Clark C, et al. The Consortium to Establish a Registry for Alzheimer's Disease CERAD: Part IV. Rates of cognitive change in longitudinal assessment of probable Alzheimer's disease. Neurology 1993;43:2457-65.

40. Haupt M, Pollman S, Kurz A. Symptom progression in AD: relation to onset of age and familial aggregation. Results of a longitudinal study. Acta Neurol Scand 1993;88:349-53.

41. Lucca U, Comeli M, Tettamanti M, Tiraboschi P, Spagnoli A. Rate of progression and prognostic factors in Alzheimer's disease: a prospective study. J Am Geriatr Soc 1993;41:45-9.

42. Lawlor BA, Ryan TM, Schmeidler J, Mohs RC, Davies KI. Clinical symptoms associated with age at onset in Alzheimer's disease. Am J Psychiatry 1994;151:1646-9.

43. Piccini C, Bracco L, Falcini M, Pracucci G, Amaducci L. Natural history of Alzheimer's disease: prognostic value of plateaux. J Neurol Sci 1995;131:177-82.

44. De Carli C, Haxby JV, Gillette JA, Teichberg D, Rapoport SI, Shapiro MB. Longitudinal changes in lateral ventricular volume in patients with dementia of the Alzheimer type. Neurology 1992;42:2029-36.

45. Jobst KA, Smith AD, Szarmari M, et al. Rapidly progressing atrophy of medial temporal lobe in Alzheimer's disease. Lancet 1994;343:829-30.

46. Fox NC, Freeborough PA, Rossor MN. Visualisation and quantification of rates of atrophy in Alzheimer's disease. Lancet 1996;348:94-7.

47. Rosen WWG, Mohs RC, Davis KL. A new rating scale for Alzheimer's disease. Am J Psychiatry 1984;141:1356-64.

48. Stern RG, Mohs RC, Davidson M, et al. A longitudinal study of Alzheimer's disease: measurement, rate and predictors of cognitive deterioration. Am J Psychiatry 1994;151:390-6.

49. Doraiswamy PM, Bieber F, Kaiser L, Krishnan KR, Reuning-Scherer J, Gulanski B. The Alzheimer's disease assessment scale: pattern and predictors of baseline cognitive performance in multicentre Alzheimer's disease trials. Neurology 1997;48:1511-17.

50. Albert SM, Sano M, Marder K, et al. Participation in clinical trials and long-term outcomes in Alzheimer's disease. Neurology 1997;49:38-43.

51. Heyman A, Wilkinson WE, Hurwitz BJ, et al. Early onset Alzheimer's disease: clinical predictors of institutionalization and death. Neurology 1987;37:980-4.

52. Jacobs D, Sano M, Marder K, et al. Age at onset of Alzheimer's disease: relation to pattern of cognitive dysfunction and rate of decline. Neurology 1994;44:1215-20.

53. Chui HC, Lyness SA, Sobel E, Schneider LS. Extrapyramidal signs and psychiatric symptoms predict faster cognitive decline in Alzheimer's disease. Arch Neurol 1994;51:676-81.

54. Koss E, Edland S, Fillenbaum G. Clinical and neuropsychological differences between patients with earlier and late onset of Alzheimer's disease: a CERAD analysis, part XII. Neurology 1996; 46:136-41.

55. Huff FJ, Growdon JH, Corkin S, Rosen TJ. Age at onset and rate of progression of Alzheimer's disease. J Am Geriatr Soc 1987;35:27-30.

56. Drachman DA, O'Donnell BF, Lew RA, Swearee JM. The prognosis of Alzheimer's disease. 'How far' rather than 'how fast' best predicts the course. Arch Neurol 1990;47:851-6.

57. Bracco L, Gallato R, Grigoletto F, et al. Factors affecting course and survival in Alzheimer's disease. A nine-year longitudinal study. Arch Neurol 1994;51:1213-19.

58. Duara R, Barker WW, Lopez-Alberola R, et al. Alzheimer's disease: interaction of apolipoprotein E genotype, family history of dementia, gender, education, ethnicity and age of onset. Neurology 1996;46:1575-9.

59. Poirer J, Delisli MC, Quirion R, et al. Apolipoprotein E4 allele as a predictor of cholinergic deficits and treatment outcome in Alzheimer's disease. Proc Natl Acad Sci USA 1995;92:12260-4.

60. Paganini-Hill A, Henderson VW. Estrogen replacement therapy and risk of Alzheimer's disease. Arch Intern Med 1996;156:2213-17.

61. Kawas C, Resnick S, Morrison A, et al. A prospective study of estrogen replacement therapy and the risk of developing Alzheimer's disease: the Baltimore Longitudinal Study of Aging. Neurology 1997;48:1517-21.

62. Baldereschi M, Di Carlo A, Grigoletto F. Estrogen replacement therapy and Alzheimer's disease in the Italian longitudinal study on aging. Neurology, in press.

63. Schneider LS, Farlow MR, Henderson VW, Pogoda JM. Effects of estrogen replacement therapy on response to tacrine in patients with Alzheimer's disease. Neurology 1996;46:1580-4.

64. Birge ST. Is there a role for estrogen replacement therapy in the prevention and treatment of dementia? J Am Geriatr Soc 1996;44:865-70.

65. Zhang M, Katzman R, Salmon D, et al. The prevalence of dementia and Alzheimer's disease in Shanghai, China: impact of age, gender and education. An Neurol 1990;11:601-7.

66. Bonaiuto S, Rocca WA, Lippi A, et al. Impact of education and occupation on the prevalence of Alzheimer's disease (AD) and multi-infarct dementia (MID) in Appignano, Macerata Province, Italy. Neurology 1990;40(suppl 1):346-7.

67. Fratiglioni L, Grut M, Forsell Y, et al. Prevalence of Alzheimer's disease and other dementias in an urban elderly population: relationship with age, sex and education. Neurology 1990;41:1886-92.

68. Katzman R. Education and the prevalence of dementia and Alzheimer's disease. Neurology 1993;43:13-20.

69. Friedland RP. Epidemiology, education and the ecology of Alzheimer's disease. Neurology 1993;43:246-9.

70. Stern Y, Alexander GE, Prohovnik I, Mayeux R. Inverse relationship of education and parietotemporal perfusion deficit in Alzheimer's disease. Ann Neurol 1992;32:371-5.

71. Coob JL, Wolf PA, Au R, White R, D'Agostino RB. The effect of education on the incidence of dementia and Alzheimer's disease in the Framingham Study. Neurology 1995;45:1707-21.

72. Chui HC, Lee Teng E, Henderson V, Moy AC. Clinical subtypes of dementia of the Alzheimer type. Neurology 1985;35:1544-50.

73. Stern Y, Albert M, Brandt J, et al. Utility of extrapyramidal signs and psychosis as predictors of cognitive and functional decline, nursing home administration, and death in Alzheimer's disease. Prospective analyses from the Predictors Study. Neurology 1994;44:2300-7.

74. McKheith IG, Galasko D, Kosaka K, et al. Consensus guidelines for the clinical and pathologic diagnosis of dementia with Lewy bodies (DLB): report of the consortium on DLB international workshop. Neurology 1996;47:1113-24.

75. Mann UM, Mohr E, Gearing M, Chase TN. Heterogeneity in Alzheimer's disease: progression rate segregated by distinct neuropsychological and

cerebral metabolic profiles. J Neurol Neurosurg Psychiatry 1992;55:956-9.

76. Butters MA, Lopez OL, Becker JT. Focal temporal lobe dysfunction in probable Alzheimer's disease predicts a slow rate of cognitive decline. Neurology 1996;46:687-92.

77. Jorm AF. Subtypes of Alzheimer's dementia: a conceptual analysis and critical review. Psychol Med 1985;15:543-53.

78. Yesavage JA, Brooks JO III, Taylor J, Tinklenberg J. Development of aphasia, apraxia and agnosia and decline in Alzheimer's disease. Am J Psychiatry 1993;150:742-7.

79. Heyman A, Peterson B, Fillenbaum G, Pieper C. The Consortium to Establish a Registry for Alzheimer's Disease (CERAD). Part XIV: demographic and clinical predictors of survival in patients with Alzheimer's disease. Neurology 1996;46:656-60.

80. Kraemer HC, Tinklenberg J, Ysavage JA. 'How far' vs 'How fast' in Alzheimer's disease. The question revisited. Arch Neurol 1994;551:275-9.

81. National Institute of Aging/Alzheimer's Association Working group. Consensus Statement. Apolipoprotein E genotype in Alzheimer's disease. Lancet 1996;347:1091-5.

82. Farlow MR. Alzheimer's disease: clinical implications of the apolipoprotein E genotype. Neurology 1997;48(suppl 6):S30-4.

83. Petersen RC, Smith GE, Ivnik RJ, et al. Apolipoprotein status as a predictor of the development of Alzheimer's disease in memory-impaired individuals. JAMA 1995;273:1274-8.

84. Tierney MC, Szalai JP, Snow WG, et al. A prospective study of the clinical utility of ApoE genotyping the prediction of outcome in patients with memory impairment. Neurology 1996;46:149-54.

85. Kurtz A, Egensperger R, Haupt M, et al. Apolipoprotein E $\epsilon 4$ allele, cognitive decline, and deterioration of everyday performance in Alzheimer's disease. Neurology 1996;47:440-3.

86. Growden JH, Locascio JJ, Corkin S, Gomez-Isla T, Hyman BT. Apolipoprotein genotype does not influence rates of cognitive decline in Alzheimer's disease. Neurology 1996;47:444-8.

87. Basun H, Grut M, Winbald B, Lannfelt L. ApoE epsilon 4 allele and disease progression in patients with late-onset AD. Neurosci Lett 1995;183:32-4.

88. Frisoni GB, Govoni S, Geroldi C. Gene dose of the $\epsilon 4$ allele of apolipoprotein E and disease progression in sporadic late-onset Alzheimer's disease. Ann Neurol 1995;37:596-604.

89. Wolfe N, Reed B, Eberling JL, Jagust WJ. Temporal lobe perfusion on single photon emission computed tomography predicts the rate of cognitive decline in Alzheimer's disease. Arch Neurol 1995;52:257-62.

90. Lopez OL, Becker JT, Rezek D, et al. Preliminary analysis of the consequences of cerebral white matter lesions in probable Alzheimer's disease. Arch Neurol 1992;49:828-34.

91. Marder K, Bello J, Bello K, et al. Progression of Alzheimer's disease over four years in patients with silent stroke. Ann Neurol 1994;36:269.

92. Berg L, Miller JP, Baty J, Rubin EH, Figiel G. Mild senile dementia of Alzheimer type 4. Evaluation of intervention. Ann Neurol 1992;31:242-9.

93. Clipp EC, Moore MJ. Caregiver time use: an outcome measure in clinical trials research on Alzheimer's disease. Clin Pharmacol Ther 1995;58:228-36.

Outcome variables in research and in practice

Michel Panisset and Serge Gauthier

This chapter explores ways in which to adapt the cumbersome testing performed within randomized clinical trials to the world of the regular clinic attended by physicians who are not necessarily specialized in memory disorders but are likely to encounter a number of demented patients. This exercise is highly needed with the general availability of newly released medications for the treatment of Alzheimer's disease (AD).

Introduction

AD is a relentlessly progressive disease with cognitive, functional and behavioral changes over time. The initial manifestations are usually short-term memory loss and executive function impairment. Depression is a frequent feature of the early stages. Behavioral changes tend to occur in the middle stages, whereas motor signs become a problem in the later stages. Most therapeutic trials have dealt with mild to moderate stages of the disease.

In selecting outcome variables, one needs to take into account the natural evolution of the disease and how it can be modified with various interventions.

Preclinical diagnosis

The preclinical stages of AD are still impossible to accurately diagnose. Genetic testing using the allele epsilon 4 of apolipoprotein E poses significant ethical problems, not to mention the consequences on future insurability, and on the psychological reaction of the subjects and their relatives.[1] The use of specific neuropsychological tests[2] in conjunction with structural[3] or metabolic[4] imaging could help to detect AD in genetically predisposed individuals. Such a strategy will be of importance when a stabilizing or preventing therapy becomes available.

Cognitive deficits

The natural cognitive deterioration of AD has been extensively studied.[5] A model of this involution has been proposed using the Mini-Mental State Examination (MMSE) scores.[6,7] This model offers a limited perspective on a very complex syndrome because of the relative narrowness of the domain covered by the MMSE.[8] Most of the instruments aimed at measuring cognitive deficits in AD have targeted the early stages of the disease, i.e. soon after the diagnosis is made. The MMSE and the cognitive component of the Alzheimer Disease Assessment Scale (ADAS-Cog)[9] have been used extensively, but these tests lack sensitivity in subjects with a high level of performance. Tests that target executive functions are likely to be more useful in this group.

The MMSE is widely used either as a screening test or as a measure of disease severity. It is simple to administer and takes about 10–15 min, so it is suitable in the context of a busy practice. The effects of education and age on the MMSE score have been extensively studied.[10] On average, there is a yearly deterioration of three points.[11] The modified MMSE or 3MS[12] contains more executive questions, is more balanced for verbal and non-verbal material, and therefore appears more sensitive to early changes.

The ADAS-Cog has been the neuropsychological test predominantly used in North American therapeutic trials. It consists of a battery of neuropsychological tests for different cognitive functions. Included are measures of verbal memory (learning, free recall and recognition), naming, comprehension, constructional praxis, ideational praxis and orientation, and examination of spontaneous speech. The battery comes to a single score with a maximum of 70 points and is administered in about 45 min. Its applicability to the regular clinical setting is limited by the time factor. Additions of attention and executive tasks to the ADAS-Cog could widen its applicability to earlier stages of dementia.[13]

The Consortium to Establish a Registry for Alzheimer's Disease (CERAD) neuropsychological battery is a good alternative which takes about the same time and includes executive tasks such as categorical verbal fluency and the Trail Making Test.[14] The Mattis Dementia Rating Scale[15] covers the domains of attention, initiation and perseveration, construction, conceptualization, and memory. It takes 30–45 min for a demented subject and has a high internal reliability.[16] The Repeatable Battery for the Assessment of Dementia[17] and the Cognitive Drug Research Computerized Battery[18] would be also sensitive in early disease.

Other tests include the Mental Status Checklist,[19] the Geriatric Interpersonal Rating Scale,[20] the Short Portable Mental Status Questionnaire[21] and the Short Blessed.[22] These are all short tests that vary slightly in content from the MMSE.

In the more advanced stages of the disease, a small number of tests is now available. The Severe Impairment Battery (SIB)[23,24] has been shown to measure cognition when other more conventional tests have reached a floor effect. Nine cognitive domains can be assessed and scored independently, including language, visual perception, memory, attention, social interaction, orientation, praxis and construction. It is reliable and sensitive to change over time.

Severity scales

A number of scales allow the staging of AD through its course, the best known being the Global Deterioration Scale (GDS), the Clinical Dementia Rating Scale (CDR) and the Functional Rating Scale (FRS).

The CDR[25] measures performance in six domains: memory, orientation, judgment and problem-solving, community affairs, home and hobbies, and personal care. The scores in each of the domains are summarized into a global score from 0 (no dementia) to 5 (severe dementia). Its reliability has been established and it has been used longitudinally and against autopsy.[26-28] The FRS uses the same system but has added two other domains: language and behavior.[29]

The Brief Cognitive Rating Scale (BCRS) is a semi-structured questionnaire[30] which assesses attention, concentration, recent and past memory, orientation, speech, praxis, calculation, self-care, psychomotor function, mood and behavior. The GDS[31] was derived from the BCRS and provides a description of the key features of AD progression on a seven-point scale.

The Hierarchic Dementia Scale has been shown to be sensitive at both ends of the spectrum of AD.[32] It measures memory, language, praxis, gnosis and motor behavior and includes tests of primitive reflexes.

The Cambridge Mental Disorders of the Eldely Examination (CAMDEX) measures physical and mental health, cognition, interviewer observation of behavior, physical examination, laboratory and radiographic tests, medications, additional comments and a structured interview of an informant.[33]

Activities of daily living assessment

The activities of daily living (ADL) are becoming increasingly important as outcome variables in research. Some governmental agencies even require an improvement in ADL to be correlated with the cognitive improvement (see Chapter 5). Measures of ADL are useful in translating changes on a cognitive scale into the real world (ecology of the changes). Most available ADL scales measure features that are problematic in moderate or moderately severe stages of the disease. Also, existing scales may not be specific to AD, and may be gender-biased (older men, as a rule, do not participate in household chores). The Functional Activity Questionnaire (FAQ),[34] the Disability Assessment in Dementia (DAD),[35] the PSMS-IADL,[36] the IDDD,[37] and the NOSGER[38] are amongst the available tests.

The FAQ is simple and quick to administer, which makes it particularly suitable for general clinical practice settings. It is most appropriate for the early stages of the disease. The PSMS-IADL scale is well known in geriatric practice and is likely to be sensitive in moderate stages of the disease.

The DAD has been developed to measure ADL impairment specifically in AD. It is a 40-item questionnaire on instrumental and self-care activities. It is a more complex tool compared to previous scales, in that it provides more information on the actual ability of the subjects and helps in differentiating between problems at the levels of the planning and the execution of the action. The DAD adequately measures ADL through the early and intermediate stages of AD and has the advantage of not showing a gender bias.

Behavioral changes

Behavioral changes are probably responsible for most of the institutionalization and most caregiver burnouts. The NeuroPsychiatric Invention (NPI)[39] and the Behave-AD[40] are the two most widely used scales.

The Sandoz Clinical Assessment Geriatric[41] contains items that are mainly focused on mood, depression, anxiety, irritability, and emotional lability.

The Behave-AD helps in the assessment of paranoia, delusions, hallucinations, anxieties and other behavioral problems often encountered with demented patients.

The NPI is based on a structured interview with the caregiver. It assesses 12 types of neuropsychiatric disturbances including delusions, hallucinations, dysphoria, anxiety, agitation, euphoria, apathy, irritability, disinhibition, aberrant motor behavior, night-time behavior disturbance and appetite and eating behaviors. Each disturbance is screened with one question and more precisely characterized with the help of subquestions when present. The frequency is scored on a four-point scale and the severity on a three-point scale. The caregiver distress is also rated for each one of the symptoms. A total NPI score as well as subscores for each symptom and for caregiver distress are available.[39,42,43] The NPI has been shown to be reliable and valid.

Holistic impression

There is a place for a global impression of change in the particular setting of a therapeutic trial and in general practice. This measure has been systematized in study protocols as suggested by the FDA. Many versions of the Clinical Global Impression of Change (CGIC) have appeared.[44] The scale usually requires an interview with the patients and with the caregiver so that the clinician can assess whether the patient under treatment has improved his or her level of functioning in everyday life. It is usually scored on a seven-point range of marked, moderate or mild improvement or deterioration, and no change. Global scoring scales such as the FRS, the CDR and the GDS-FAST system have supplemented the CGIC in order to improve its reliability. The use of the CGIC provides an ecological approach. The most widely used CGIC has been developed by the Alzheimer's Disease Cooperative Study (ADCS).[45]

A novel approach is to target the symptoms that one would particularly like to see improve.[46] This Goal Attainment Scaling (GAS) is an individualized measurement approach that accommodates multiple individual patient goals, and has a scoring system which allows for comparisons between patients. It has been shown to be more sensitive to change compared to other measures of disability.

Milestones

Using milestones of dementia is another way of assessing the evolution of dementia. This method has been recently used in the study by Sano et al.[47] They examined the effect of selegiline, tocopherol and placebo in moderately demented patients, and used mortality, institutionalization and going from a CDR of 2 to a CDR of 3 as measure of progression. Other milestones that could be used early in AD are the inability to manage financial affairs, to drive a car, to cook with a recipe, to go out alone, or to be left at home alone, or the development of hallucinations or of incontinence, but these may show significant interindividual variance.

From therapeutic trials to office practice

The therapeutic trials require a team of clinicians to administer these scales and a large amount of time from patients, caregivers and raters. Now that medications are becoming available for regular use, it becomes important that we have tools that are usable in everyday practice. Since many patients will be seen by their general practitioners, instruments will need to be adapted for their practice. Indeed, since not all patients will improve on AD medications, it is necessary for the physicians to determine whether a patient is a responder or not.

Since it may be difficult to conduct a systematic interview as dictated by the

CGIC, one could use scales such as the CDR or the FRS as a frame to explore different cognitive, functional and behavioral domains. These scales will have to be supplemented with personal notes, since their scoring systems may not be sensitive enough to translate the changes observed by the caregivers. These scales can be supplemented by a target symptom list. A more objective measure of the cognition and of the level of ADL should also be included in follow-up visits. Our own preference go to the 3MS or the MMSE, and the FAQ or the DAD. This battery of scales should be appropriate to follow patients on the available medications indicated for the treatment of AD and appears to be a good balance between time and face value.

References

1. Post SG, Whitehouse PJ, Binstock RH, et al. The clinical introduction of genetic testing for Alzheimer disease. An ethical perspective. JAMA 1997;277:832-6.

2. Reid W, Broe G, Creasey H, et al. Age at onset and pattern of neuropsychological impairment in mild early-stage Alzheimer disease. Arch Neurol 1996;53:1056-61.

3. Kaye JA, Swihart T, Howieson D, et al. Volume loss of the hippocampus and temporal lobe in healthy elderly persons destined to develop dementia. Neurology 1997;48:1297-304.

4. Reiman WM, Caselli RJ, Yun LS, et al. Preclinical evidence of Alzheimer's disease in persons homozygous for the E4 allele for apolipoprotein E. N Engl J Med 1996;334:752-8.

5. Panisset M, Stern Y. Prognostic factors. In: Gauthier S, ed. Clinical diagnosis and management of Alzheimer's disease. London: Martin Dunitz Ltd, 1996:129-39.

6. Folstein MF, Folstein SE, McHugh PR. 'Mini Mental State': a practical method for grading the cognitive state of patients for the clinician. J Psychiatr Res 1975;12:189-98.

7. Brooks JO, Kraemer HC, Tanke ED, Yesavage JA. The methodology of studying decline in Alzheimer's disease. J Am Geriatr Soc 1993;41:623-8.

8. Goldblum MC, Tzortizis C, Michot JL, Panisset M, Boller F. Language impairment and rate of cognitive decline in Alzheimer's disease. Dementia 1994;5:334-8.

9. Rosen WG, Mohs RC, Davis KL. A new rating scale for Alzheimer's disease. Am J Psychiatr 1984;141:1356-64.

10. Bleeker ML, Bolla-Wilson K, Kawas C, Agnew J. Age-specific norms for the Mini Mental State Exam. Neurology 1988;38:1565-8.

11. Salmon DP, Thal IJ, Butters N, Heindel WC. Longitudinal evaluation of dementia of the Alzheimer type: a comparison of 3 standardized mental status examinations. Neurology 1990;40:1225-30.

12. Teng EL, Chui CH. The modified Mini-Mental State (3MS). J Clin Psychiatry 1987;48:314-18.

13. Mohs RC, Knopman D, Petersen RC et al. Development of cognitive instruments for use in clinical trials of antidementia drugs: additions to the Alzheimer's disease assessment scale that broaden its scope. Alzheimer Dis Assoc Disord 1997;11(suppl 2):S13-21.

14. Morris JC, Heyman A, Mohs RC et al. The Consortium to Establish a Registry for Alzheimer's Disease. Part I. Clinical and neuropsychological assessment of Alzheimer's disease. Neurology 1989;39:1159-65.

15. Mattis S. Dementia rating scale professional manual. Odessa: Psychological Assessment Resources, 1988.

16. Gardner R Jr, Oliver-Munoz S, Fisher L, Empting L. Mattis Dementia Rating Scale: internal reliability study using a diffusely impaired population. J Clin Neuropsychol 1981;3:271-5.

17. Randolph C. Repeatable battery for the assessment of dementia (BRAD). New York: Psychological Corporation, in press.

18. Wesnes K. A fully automated psychometric test battery for human psychopharmacology. In: Abstracts of the IVth World Congress of Biological Psychiatry. Philadelphia, 1985:153.

19. Lifshitz K. Problems in the quantitative evaluation of patients with psychoses of the senium. J Psychol 1960;49:295-303.

20. Plutchik R, Conte H, Lieberman M. Development of a scale (GIES) for the assessment of cognitive and perceptual functioning in geriatric patients. J Am Geriatr Soc 1971;19:614-23.

21. Pfeiffer E. SPMSQ: short portable mental status questionnaire. J Am Geriatr Soc 1975;23:433-41.

22. Blessed G. Tomlinson BE, Roth M. The association between qualitative measures of dementia and senile change in the cerebral grey matter of elderly subjects. Br J Psychiatry 1968;114:797-811.

23. Saxton J, McGonigle-Gibson K, Swihart A, Miller M, Boller F. Assessment of the severely impaired patients: description and validation of a new neuropsychological test battery. Psychol Assess 1990;2:298-303.

24. Panisset M, Roudier M, Saxton J, Boller F. Severe Impairment Battery: a neuropsychological battery for severely demented patients. Arch Neurol 1994;51:41-5.

25. Morris J. Clinical Dementia Rating (CDR): current version and scoring rules. Neurology 1993;43:2412-14.

26. Burke WJ, Miller P, Rubin EH, et al. Reliability of the Washington University Clinical Dementia Rating. Arch Neurol 1988;54:3-32.

27. Morris JC, McKeel DW, Fulling K, et al. Validation of clinical diagnostic criteria for Alzheimer's disease. Ann Neurol 1988;24:17-22.

28. Galasko D, Edland SD, Morris JC, et al. The Consortium to Establish a Registry for Alzheimer's Disease (CERAD). Part XI. Clinical milestones in patients with Alzheimer's disease followed over three years. Neurology 1995;45:1451-5.

29. Feldman H, Schulzer M, Wang S, et al. The Functional Rating Scale (FRS) in Alzheimer's disease assessment: a longitudinal study. In: Iqbal K, Mortimer J, Winbald B, Wisiewski H, eds. Research advances in Alzheimer's Disease and related disorders. Chichester: John Wiley, 1995:235-41.

30. Reisberg B, Ferris SH. Brief Cognitive Rating Scale (BCRS). Psychopharmacol Bull 1988;24:629-36.

31. Reisberg B, Ferris SH, DeLeon MJ, et al. The global deterioration scale for assessment of primary degenerative dementia. Am J Psychiatry 1982;139:1136-9.

32. Cole M, Dastoor DP. A new approach to the measurement of dementia. Psychosomatics 1987;28:298-304.

33. Roth M. The Cambridge Mental Disorders of the Elderly Examination with special reference to its use in the diagnosis of mild or early dementia. In: Canal N, Hachinski VC, McKhann G, Franceschi M, eds. Guidelines for drug trials in memory disorders. New York: Raven Press, 1993;39:219-34.

34. Pfeffer RI, Kurosaki TT, Harrah CH, et al. Measurement of functional activities in older adults in the community. J Gerontol 1982;37:323-9.

35. Gauthier L, Gauthier S, Gélinas I et al. Assessment of functioning and ADL. In: Abstract Book of the 6th Congress of the IPA. Berlin, September, 1993.

36. Lawton MP, Brody EM. Asssessment of older people: self-maintaining and instrumental activities of daily living. Gerontologist 1969;9:176-86.

37. Teunisse S, Derix MM, van Crevel H. Assessing the severity of dementia. Patient and caregiver. Arch Neurol 1991;48:274-7.

38. Spiegel R, Brunner C, Ermini-Funfschilling D, et al. A new behavioral assessment scale for geriatric out- and in-patients: the NOSGER (Nurses' Observational Scale for Geriatric Patients). J Am Geriatr Soc 1991;39:339-47.

39. Cummings JL, Mega M, Gray K, et al. The Neuropsychiatric Inventory: comprehensive assessment of psychopathology in dementia. Neurology 1994;44:2308-14.

40. Reisberg B, Borenstein J, Salob SP, et al. Behavioral symptoms in Alzheimer's disease: phenomenology and treatment. J Clin Psychiatry 1987;48:9-15.

41. Shader RI, Harmatz JS, Salzman C. A new scale for clinical assessment in geriatric populations: Sandoz Clinical Assessment-Geriatric (SGAG). J Am Geriatr Soc 1974;22:107-13.

42. Cummings JL. The Neuropsychiatric Inventory: assessing psychopathology in dementia patients. Neurology 1997;48(suppl):S10-16.

43. Mega M, Cummings JL, Fiorello T et al. The spectrum of behavioral changes in Alzheimer's disease. Neurology 1996;46:130-5.

44. Rockwood K, Morris JC. Global staging measures in dementia. In: Gauthier S, ed. Clinical diagnosis and management of Alzheimer's disease. London: Martin Dunitz Ltd, 1996:141-50.

45. Schneider LS, Obin JT, Doody RS, et al. Validity and reliability of the Alzheimer's Disease Cooperative Study: Clinical Global Impression of Change. Alzheimer Dis Assoc Disord 1997;11(suppl 2):S22-32.

46. Rockwood K, Stolee P, Howard K, Mallery L. Use of Goal Attainment Scaling to measure treatment effects in an anti-dementia drug trial. Neuroepidemiology 1996;15:330-8.

47. Sano M, Eernesto C, Thomas RG, et al. A controlled trial of selegiline, alpha tocopherol, or both as treatment for Alzheimer's disease. N Engl J Med 1997;336:1216-22.

Trial designs

Michael Grundman and Leon J. Thal

Introduction

The focus of this chapter is phase III clinical trials for the treatment or prevention of Alzheimer's disease (AD). The purpose of such trials is to determine the efficacy of a putative treatment under conditions that are likely to exist once a drug is marketed and to assess the agent's medium- and long-term side-effects. Phase III studies are usually large, multicenter trials that are randomized and placebo-controlled, with the treatment assignment unknown to the investigator or patient (double-blind). Such trials are necessary for drug approval in many countries.

Prior to phase III clinical trials, phase I studies are conducted to determine the acute safety, tolerance and pharmacokinetics of an agent in small samples of volunteers. Following phase I, phase II studies begin to examine efficacy and assess the range of doses that may be effective. Phase II studies also extend the safety profile of the drug to include short-term adverse side-effects and further define the drug's pharmacokinetic properties.

Phase III clinical trials for AD may be conducted for a variety of indications: (1) to determine symptomatic benefit; (2) to slow apparent disease progression; or (3) to delay the onset of the clinical diagnosis of AD. Regardless of the indication, phase III trials share certain elements in common. First, the hypothesis of the study is stated explicitly. The study population is defined and an adequate sample size is calculated to provide a definitive test of the hypothesis. Treatment assignment must be random, as otherwise the investigator could influence the outcome of the trial in favor of the active agent. Study end-points are chosen which are objective and clinically meaningful. In current AD trials, demonstration of efficacy is needed on multiple end-points including at least a cognitive test instrument and a clinician's global impression under FDA guidelines. Clinical evaluations are performed blind to treatment assignment to deter potential bias in favor of the active treatment. Early phase III clinical trials for AD tended to use a cross-over design.[1-8] In a simple two-period cross-over design, every patient is treated twice, once with the active agent and once with placebo. Depending on whether the subject is assigned to treatment or placebo during the first period, the subject is then assigned the alternative treatment during the second period. The major appeal of cross-over studies is that each subject serves as his or her own control, reducing the variance contributed by between-subject differences. In a cross-over study, it is assumed that there are no carry-over effects, withdrawal effects or treatment by period interactions. Patients entering the second treatment period should return to the clinical state exhibited prior to the start of the first period. Unfortunately, period and order effects may occur, particularly if the disease progresses during the course of the trial. There is also the possibility that the investigator or patient may become unblinded at the time of cross-over. Patient dropouts are more of a problem in cross-over studies, because subjects must receive both treatments in order to provide optimal information. Small cross-over trials may not permit the statistical assumptions of the study design to be evaluated reliably.

Another study design[9,10] that has been utilized in AD trials is the 'enrichment design'. This type of clinical trial is performed in two stages. During the first stage, all participants are dose-titrated with the active drug in an attempt to identify a subgroup of potential responders and to determine optimal dosing for each subject. During the second stage, the subjects identified as potential responders in the first stage are randomized to active treatment or placebo. The non-responding subjects from the first stage are dropped from the study. Advantages of this design include the ability to determine the most effective dose during the dose titration phase and to drop non-responding subjects early. A disadvantage of this design is that all patients are exposed to the drug, making it difficult to determine true adverse event profiles. Carry-over effects may occur when patients are crossed over to placebo. Finally, it is difficult to generalize the trial results from the pre-selected patients involved in the study to Alzheimer's patients in the community.

Parallel group designs[9-18] are now more common, as some of the drawbacks of cross-over or enrichment designs for the evaluation of dementia drugs have become more widely recognized. In a parallel group design, the trial participants are divided at random into as many groups as there are treatments. The analysis of parallel group studies relies on fewer assumptions than that of cross-over designs. A disadvantage of the parallel group design is that the variability between subjects is greater than that within subjects, requiring more subjects for the same statistical power. It is also generally assumed that the randomization process will balance important prognostic factors between the treatment groups. This does not always occur. There is always the need to verify the comparability of the treatment groups, and, if necessary, perform an analysis adjusting for uneven distribution of prognostic factors.

The outcome measures chosen in phase III clinical trials of AD have traditionally been change scores between the last treatment visit and the baseline on a continuous or ordinal measurement scale, e.g. the ADAS-Cog[19] or a clinician's global impression.[20] Change scores on continuous measures have limited clinical interpretation. A specific change score on the ADAS-Cog, for example, cannot be readily understood in a clinically meaningful way. Continuous measures also suffer from lack of linearity over their entire spectrum and are susceptible to ceiling and floor effects, depending on the severity of the patient's condition. This is a problem because it is frequently assumed that the same change score on a test reflects an equal change in performance. Similarly, subjects who drop out of a clinical trial early cannot provide the correct change score needed for the statistical analysis.

Time-to-event outcomes and survival analysis have certain advantages compared to continuous measurement scales. This methodology has been used successfully in a recent clinical trial of AD.[21,22] The knowledge that a subject has survived for a certain period of time without reaching the trial end-point can be utilized in survival analyses, even if the subject is removed (censored) prior to the end of the study. Survival methods also have the capacity to include important prognostic variables other than the treatment in the analysis (e.g. using the Cox proportional hazards model) and may be used to adjust for potential baseline imbalances between the treatment groups. End-points chosen for studies with a survival design should be clinically meaningful, well recognized, unlikely to be missed and stable from subsequent recovery. Ideally, they should occur consistently as the underlying disease progresses and reflect the

magnitude of the underlying pathology. The end-points should occur frequently enough during the period of follow-up such that the results are not limited to a small minority of the population randomized. Trials using end-points that occur only infrequently after long observation periods require very large numbers of subjects in order to demonstrate a treatment effect.

Despite the advantages of discrete outcomes and survival analysis, there are some caveats. The relevance and validity of the outcome may be questioned even if the outcome is unambiguous and occurs relatively consistently (e.g. death and institutionalization).[23] Dementia is a contributing cause of death in approximately three-quarters of AD patients;[24] however, some deaths may not be related to AD (e.g. patients may die of cancer or myocardial infarction). Institutionalization, while usually related to disease severity, may be prompted by other variables, e.g. difficult behavioral problems, caregiver characteristics or the availability of a suitable nursing home. Other outcomes which are more directly related to dementia severity, such as conversion to a certain severity stage on the Clinical Dementia Rating,[25,26] or the diagnosis of AD, require clinical experience and training to ensure reliability between investigators and centers.

Symptomatic studies

The primary goal of studies involving symptomatic agents is to demonstrate improvement in core symptoms of the disease, such as memory impairment. Ideally, patients recruited to studies testing symptomatic agents should have probable AD according to the NINCDS-ADRDA criteria.[27] Trials should last for 3–6 months. In order to ensure that a clinical trial produces both a beneficial effect on core symptoms of the disease and an effect that is large enough to be recognizable by a skilled clinician, a performance-based cognitive assessment and a clinical global assessment is generally used. The cognitive assessment tool preferred most frequently is the ADAS-Cog.[19] Clinical global assessments that have been utilized include the Clinician's Interview Based Impression of Change (CIBIC) and the ADCS Clinical Global Impression of Change (ADCS-CGIC).[20,28] Assessments in other domains are frequently performed as well, including an evaluation of activities of daily living (ADL) and behavior. Among ADL scales that are currently being used are the

Physical Self-Maintenance and Instrumental Activities of Daily Living Scales,[29,30] the Progressive Deterioration Scale,[31] the Disability Assessment in Dementia[32] and the ADCS-ADL.[33] Frequently used behavioral scales include the BEHAVE-AD[34] and the Neuropsychiatric Inventory.[35]

Definitive phase III studies of symptomatic agents generally require 100–200 subjects per treatment group, depending on the assumptions involved in the power analysis. To ensure sufficient power for a trial, an estimate of the rate of progression on the ADAS-Cog for the placebo-treated subjects over the duration of the trial is required. Also required is an estimate of the mean difference in performance between the placebo and treatment groups on the ADAS-Cog that is considered clinically meaningful or that would be considered desirable to detect. Studies are often designed with 90% power in order to ensure sufficient power on both the cognitive measure and global assessment. Previously published studies reporting a symptomatic benefit in AD,[13,15,36] found a deterioration on the ADAS-Cog over 6-months of 1.4–2.0 points for the placebo-treated group. Observed differences on the ADAS-Cog for treatment versus placebo averaged between 2 and 5 points for subjects completing those trials. A mean difference between the active treatment and placebo group of at least 2.5 points is considered desirable for symptomatic trials.

In order to accelerate a drug's development, sponsors may choose to merge phases II and III. One approach is to conduct large multicenter studies to gather definitive evidence of both safety and efficacy. This entails the enrollment of large numbers of subjects to placebo and two or three widely spaced doses of the drug. Sometimes, the highest dose is used as the primary comparison with placebo. Alternatively, if there are reasons to suspect a possible U-shaped dose–response curve, the statistical significance may be made more stringent than $p = 0.05$ to account for the several planned comparisons.

Slowing decline

Clinical trials designed for agents that may slow the rate of disease progression should take into account the fact that the size of the treatment effect will be proportional to the duration of the study. The longer the study, the greater will be the absolute difference

in the outcome measure between the treatment and placebo groups (Figure 4.1). Longer trials will require fewer patients, because the treatment effect size will grow in comparison to the variability of the test itself with repeated testing. Longer trials, however, are susceptible to a greater number of dropouts. Subjects selected to participate in such trials should be medically stable in order to remain in the study for at least 1 year. The ADAS-Cog and CGIC are appropriate instruments for trials lasting up to 1 year. For trials lasting much beyond 1 year, however, the CGIC, in particular, may not be ideal because of the increasing likelihood that raters will change and the baseline examination will be increasingly difficult to recall. A previously published trial found a deterioration rate on the ADAS-Cog of 7.0 points per year for the placebo-treated group.[14] Based on this estimate, a 1-year trial designed to detect a 50% reduction in the rate of decline requires 75–125 subjects per treatment arm. A greater number of subjects than this is needed if detection of a smaller treatment difference is desired.

Additional trial design elements may help to determine whether a putative therapeutic agent exerts a symptomatic effect

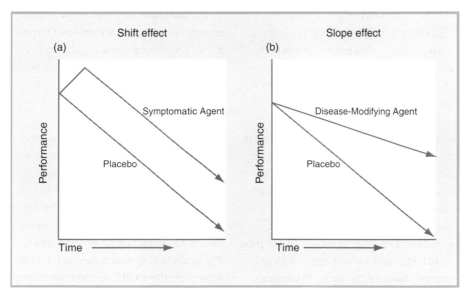

Figure 4.1
Symptomatic agents result in a short-term improvement without altering the underlying slope of deterioration (A). Disease-modifying agents, by slowing disease progression, reduce the slope (B). Note that the treatment benefit increases over time with disease-modifying agents but remains constant with symptomatic agents.

or slows the rate of progression of the disease (shift effect versus slope effect) (Figure 4.1). Two trial maneuvers that have been suggested are the 'randomized start' and 'randomized withdrawal' designs (Figure 4.2). The more common approach is the 'randomized withdrawal' design (Figure 4.2A). In this design, subjects on active drug at the conclusion of the trial are switched to placebo, while those on placebo at the trial's conclusion remain on placebo. Subjects who took the active drug during the trial should lose efficacy over time, and drift toward the placebo group after being placed on placebo, if the drug only has a symptomatic effect. Such a pattern was observed in the 30-week donepezil trial.[36] In the 'randomized start' design (Figure 4.2B), one group of subjects is randomized to placebo first, followed by the active drug, while another group is randomized to the active drug and remains on the active drug throughout

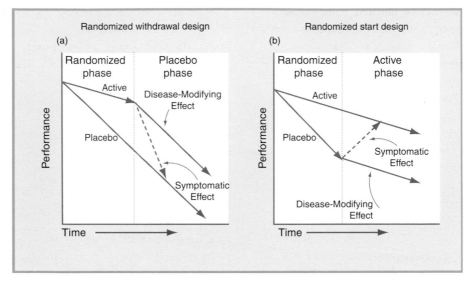

Figure 4.2
Two maneuvers are illustrated which may help to differentiate symptomatic from disease-modifying agents. In both trial designs, subjects are randomized to active drug or placebo in the first phase. During the second phase (to the right of the dotted line), all subjects are placed on placebo in the randomized withdrawal design (A) or on active drug in the randomized start design (B). The treatment benefit attributable to the active drug in the first phase is maintained in the second phase (the lines remain apart) if the agent modifies the underlying disease but not if the effect is purely symptomatic.

the trial. If the active drug has only symptomatic effects, placebo-treated patients placed on the active drug should approach the performance of those who were taking the active drug from the beginning of the trial. Alternatively, if there is a true slowing in the rate of progression such that a structural change occurs in the brains of the actively treated subjects over the course

of the trial, the placebo-treated patients who are newly placed on the active drug will not be able to catch up.[37]

Prevention studies

AD is thought to be characterized by a preclinical period during which prevention of disease symptoms may be possible.[38] The first pathologic changes of

AD may be initiated in the decades prior to the onset of clinical symptoms through genetic, traumatic, anoxic or possibly other events. It is likely that aging promotes the disease process. Clinical symptoms appear when the pathology and synaptic loss reach a critical threshold. If this model is correct, effective slowing of the disease in its incipient stage should prove more advantageous than the current approach of treating symptoms late in the course of the disease.

A recently completed clinical trial of selegiline and vitamin E found that disease milestones could be delayed by antioxidants. This suggests that the rate of progression of the disease may be slowed.[21] The primary objective of the study was to determine whether vitamin E or selegiline could delay functional decline and death. The trial enrolled patients with moderately severe disease in a double-blind, placebo-controlled, parallel group, factorial design, multicenter trial. Patients were randomly assigned to receive either vitamin E (2000 IU daily), selegiline (10 mg daily), the combination of selegiline and vitamin E, or placebo. The primary outcome measure was the time to reach one of the following endpoints: institutionalization, loss of basic

ADL, severe dementia (defined by a Clinical Dementia Rating of 3), or death. The results were analyzed using survival analysis. There were significant reductions in the risk of reaching the primary outcome with vitamin E, selegiline or the combined treatment. No evidence was found of additional improvement with the combined treatment over either treatment alone.

Vitamin E and selegiline as well as other putative disease-modifying agents that may block critical pathogenic pathways (e.g. estrogen, coenzyme Q, idebenone, nerve growth factor (NGF) agonists, COX2 inhibitors, anti-amyloid agents) are or will be undergoing clinical testing to prevent dementia in the near future. As these agents enter dementia prevention trials, it might be more efficient and cost-effective to test them in minimally symptomatic subjects with mild cognitive impairment (MCI) rather than in normal subjects. Subjects with MCI are characterized by memory complaints and consistent forgetfulness, with little if any impairment in other cognitive domains or ADL.[39] They do not meet DSM-IV criteria for dementia[40] or NINCDS-ADRDA criteria for probable AD.[27] Many MCI subjects are likely to be in a relatively early phase of the disease process and may have neuropathologic features consistent with early AD. They are at increased risk for progressing to a clinical diagnosis of AD within a few years. It is estimated that a clinical trial to prevent dementia in subjects with MCI will require 3 years of follow-up and several hundred subjects. Alternatively, a large-scale, randomized, clinical trial to prevent dementia in normal elderly subjects is estimated to require approximately 5000–8000 subjects and involve 5 or more years of follow-up. An MCI trial is estimated to cost only a fraction of that which a primary prevention trial in normal elderly subjects would cost. Once an agent is proven safe and effective in subjects with MCI, it might then be tested in larger prevention trials for longer time intervals to extend the generalizability of the findings to cognitively normal individuals.

The time required for subjects with MCI to develop a clinical diagnosis of AD has been estimated by the ADCS.[41] The cumulative incidence of AD was 31% at 2 years and 44% at 3 years. An increase in the conversion rate might be achieved by recruiting only MCI patients with documented deficits on delayed recall[42–45] or by including only individuals with one or two ApoE4 alleles.[46–52] Subject enrichment of this kind might improve the efficiency of the study and reduce the number of subjects needed.

As noted, a more costly but more general clinical trial approach to dementia prevention is a primary prevention trial in healthy, elderly individuals without any evidence of cognitive impairment. A primary prevention trial has the capacity to intervene in the disease process even prior to the development of MCI. Such a trial[53] began in 1996 (the Women's Health Initiative—Memory Study). It is an ancillary study to the Women's Health Initiative (WHI). The hypothesis being tested is that the development of dementia will be delayed in women who receive hormone therapy as compared to placebo. The study design calls for 39 WHI clinical centers across the USA to recruit approximately 8300 women between the ages of 65 and 79 over a 2-year period. Participants will be followed annually for 6–9 years. Hysterectomized and non-hysterectomized women are randomized to hormone replacement therapy (estrogen alone for women without a uterus or estrogen plus medroxyprogesterone for women with a uterus) or placebo. The screening process for dementia is staged in order to minimize patient and staff burden and cost. Initial cognitive assessment is performed using a Modified Mini-Mental State Examination.[54] Women scoring below a predetermined cut-off receive a more extensive neuropsychological test battery. Subjects suspected of developing dementia undergo a neuropsychiatric evaluation. A clinician then diagnoses the patient with probable dementia, MCI, or no dementia, based on this information. Women diagnosed with probable dementia undergo laboratory tests to classify the type of dementia (e.g. probable AD) and to rule out reversible causes. Survival analysis methods will be used to describe the estimated time to dementia and to compare the rate of conversion to dementia between the estrogen and placebo groups.

Phase IV studies

In light of the approval of two anti-dementia drug treatments and the success of the selegiline and vitamin E study, a number of new experimental designs are possible: (1) comparison of two putative symptomatic drugs in a direct comparison of efficacy; (2) combination of a putative symptomatic drug with a putative disease-modifying drug (a recent study, for example, found that subjects receiving estrogen therapy might be better responders to cholinesterase inhibitor therapy[55]); (3) combination of symptomatic drugs (e.g. the combination of a cholinesterase inhibitor with a cholinergic agonist); or (4) combinations of drugs designed to slow the rate of progression through different mechanisms.

Trials performed in specific population subgroups may also be helpful in understanding the pathogenic pathways involved in AD. Examples include trials in: (1) older or younger populations; (2) suspected Lewy body patients; (3) patients at different stages of disease severity; or (4) patients with defined mutations (e.g. the presenilins or amyloid precursor protein) or specific genotypes (e.g. ApoE4 homozygotes). There is some evidence that the ApoE genotype may influence responsiveness to drug treatment.[52,56] Other questions that may be of interest in phase IV studies include the long-term effects of a putative therapeutic agent on nursing home placement and mortality[57] and its pharmacoeconomic impact.[58]

References

1. Summers WK, Majovski LV, Marsh GM, Tachiki K, Kling A. Oral tetrahydroaminoacridine in long-term treatment of senile dementia, Alzheimer type. N Engl J Med 1986;315:1241-5.

2. Stern Y, Sano M, Mayeux R. Effects of oral physostigmine in Alzheimer's disease. Ann Neurol 1987;22:306-10.

3. Stern Y, Sano M, Mayeux R. Long-term administration of oral physostigmine in Alzheimer's disease. Neurology 1988;38:1837-41.

4. Penn RD, Martin EM, Wilson RS, Fox JH, Savoy SM. Intraventricular bethanechol infusion for Alzheimer's disease: results of double-blind and escalating-dose trials. Neurology 1988;38:219-22.

5. Blass JP, Gleason P, Brush D, DiPonte P, Thaler H. Thiamine and Alzheimer's disease. A pilot study. Arch Neurol 1988;45:833-5.

6. Mohr E, Schlegel J, Fabbrini G, et al. Clonidine treatment of Alzheimer's disease. Arch Neurol 1989;46:376-8.

7. Henderson VW, Roberts E, Wimer C, et al. Multicenter trial of naloxone in Alzheimer's disease. Ann Neurol 1989;25:404-6.

8. Gauthier S, Bouchard R, Lamontagne A, et al. Tetrahydroaminoacridine-lecithin combination treatment in patients with intermediate-stage Alzheimer's disease. Results of a Canadian double-blind, crossover, multicenter study. N Engl J Med 1990;322:1272-6.

9. Davis KL, Thal LJ, Gamzu ER, et al. A double-blind, placebo-controlled multicenter study of tacrine for Alzheimer's disease. The Tacrine Collaborative Study Group. N Engl J Med 1992;327:1253-9.

10. Thal LJ, Schwartz G, Sano M, et al. A multicenter double-blind study of controlled-release physostigmine for the treatment of symptoms secondary to Alzheimer's disease. Physostigmine Study Group. Neurology 1996;47:1389-95.

11. Farlow M, Gracon SI, Hershey LA, Lewis KW, Sadowsky CH, Dolan-Ureno J. A controlled trial of tacrine in Alzheimer's disease. The Tacrine Study Group. JAMA 1992;268:2523-9.

12. Burke WJ, Roccaforte WH, Wengel SP, Bayer BL, Ranno AE, Willcockson NK. L-Deprenyl in the treatment of mild dementia of the Alzheimer type: results of a 15-month trial. J Am Geriatr Soc 1993;41:1219-25.

13. Knapp MJ, Knopman DS, Solomon PR, Pendlebury WW, Davis CS, Gracon SI. A 30-week randomized controlled trial of high-dose tacrine in patients with Alzheimer's disease. The Tacrine Study Group. JAMA 1994;271:985-91.

14. Thal LJ, Carta A, Clarke WR, et al. A 1-year multicenter placebo-controlled study of acetyl-L-carnitine in patients with Alzheimer's disease. Neurology 1996;47:705-11.

15. Bodick NC, Offen WW, Levey AI, et al. Effects of xanomeline, a selective muscarinic receptor agonist, on cognitive function and behavioral symptoms in Alzheimer disease. Arch Neurol 1997;54:465-73.

16. Rogers SL, Friedhoff LT. The efficacy and safety of donepezil in patients with Alzheimer's disease: results of a US multicentre, randomized, double-blind, placebo-controlled trial. The Donepezil Study Group. Dementia 1996;7:293-303.

17. Rogers J, Kirby LC, Hempelman SR, et al. Clinical trial of indomethacin in Alzheimer's disease. Neurology 1993;43:1609-11.

18. Becker RE, Colliver JA, Markwell SJ, Moriearty PL, Unni LK, Vicari S. Double-blind, placebo-controlled study of metrifonate, an acetylcholinesterase inhibitor, for Alzheimer disease. Alzheimer Dis Assoc Disord 1996;10:124-31.

19. Rosen WG, Mohs RC, Davis KL. A new rating scale for Alzheimer's disease. Am J Psychiatry 1984;141:1356-64.

20. Schneider LS, Olin JT, Doody RS, et al. Validity and Reliability of the Alzheimer's Disease Cooperative Study–Clinical Global Impression of Change, The Alzheimer's Disease Cooperative Study. Alzheimer Dis Assoc Disord 1997;11(suppl. 2):S22-32.

21. Sano M, Ernesto C, Thomas RG, et al. A controlled trial of selegiline, alpha-tocopherol, or both as treatment for Alzheimer's disease. The Alzheimer's Disease Cooperative Study. N Engl J Med 1997;336:1216-22.

22. Sano M, Ernesto C, Klauber MR, et al. Rationale and design of a multicenter study of selegiline and alpha-tocopherol in the treatment of Alzheimer disease using novel clinical outcomes. Alzheimer's Disease Cooperative Study. Alzheimer Dis Assoc Disord 1996;10:132-40.

23. Drachman DA, Leber P. Treatment of Alzheimer's disease-searching for a breakthrough, settling for less. N Engl J Med 1997;336:1245-7.

24. Olichney JM, Hofstetter CR, Galasko D, Thal LJ, Katzman R. Death certificate reporting of dementia and mortality in an Alzheimer's disease research center cohort. J Am Geriatr Soc 1995;43:890-3.

25. Berg L. Clinical Dementia Rating (CDR). Psychopharmacol Bull 1988;24:637-9.

26. Morris JC. The Clinical Dementia Rating (CDR): current version and scoring rules. Neurology 1993;43:2412-14.

27. McKhann G, Drachman D, Folstein M, Katzman R, Price D, Stadlan EM. Clinical diagnosis of Alzheimer's disease: report of the NINCDS-ADRDA Work Group under the auspices of Department of Health and Human Services Task Force on Alzheimer's Disease. Neurology 1984;34:939-44.

28. Schneider LS, Olin JT. Clinical global impressions in Alzheimer's clinical trials. Int Psychogeriatr 1996;8:277-88; discussion 288-90.

29. Lawton MP. Scales to measure competence in everyday activities. Psychopharmacol Bull 1988;24:609-14.

30. Lawton MP, Brody EM. Assessment of older people: self-maintaining and instrumental activities of daily living. Gerontologist 1969;9:179-86.

31. DeJong R, Osterlund OW, Roy GW. Measurement of quality-of-life changes in patients with Alzheimer's disease. Clin Ther 1989;11:545-54.

32. Gélinas I, Gauthier L, Wood-dauphinee S, Gauthier S, Bellavance F, Wolfson C. Assessment of functional disability in Alzheimer's disease. CTOT Conference Suppl. 1995;62:15.

33. Galasko D, Bennett D, Sano M, et al. An inventory to assess activities of daily living for clinical trials in Alzheimer's disease, The Alzheimer's Disease Cooperative Study. Alzheimer Dis Assoc Disord 1997;11(suppl 2):S33-9.

34. Reisberg B, Borenstein J, Salob SP, Ferris SH, Franssen E, Georgotas A. Behavioral symptoms in Alzheimer's disease: phenomenology and treatment. J Clin Psychiatry 1987;48(Suppl):9-15.

35. Cummings JL, Mega M, Gray K, Rosenberg-Thompson S, Carusi DA, Gornbein J. The Neuropsychiatric Inventory: comprehensive assessment of psychopathology in dementia. Neurology 1994;44:2308-14.

36. Rogers SL, Farlour MR, Doody RS, Mohs R, Friedhoff LT. A 24-week, double-blind, placebo-controlled trial of donepezil in patients with Alzheimer's disease. Donepezil Study Group. Neurology 1998;50:136-45.

37. Leber P. Observations and suggestions on antidementia drug development. Alzheimer Dis Assoc Disord 1996;10(suppl 1):31-5.

38. Katzman R, Kawas C. The epidemiology of dementia and Alzheimer disease. In: Terry RD, Katzman R, Bick KL, eds. Alzheimer disease. New York: Raven Press, 1994: 105-19.

39. Petersen RC. Normal Aging, Mild Cognitive Impairment, and Early Alzheimer's Disease. Neurologist 1995;1:326-44.

40. American Psychiatric Association. Diagnostic and Statistical Manual of Mental Disorders, 4th edn. Washington, DC: American Psychiatric Association, 1994.

41. Grundman M, Petersen RC, Morris JC, et al. Rate of dementia of Alzheimer type (DAT) in subjects with mild cognitive impairment. The ADCS Cooperative Study. Neurology 1996;46:A403.

42. Masur DM, Sliwinski M, Lipton RB, Blau AD, Crystal HA. Neuropsychological prediction of dementia and the absence of dementia in healthy elderly persons. Neurology 1994;44:1427-32.

43. Tierney MC, Szalai JP, Snow WG, et al. Prediction of probable Alzheimer's disease in memory-impaired patients: a prospective longitudinal study. Neurology 1996;46:661-5.

44. Knopman DS, Ryberg S. A verbal memory test with high predictive accuracy for dementia of the Alzheimer type. Arch Neurol 1989;46:141–5.

45. Welsh K, Butters N, Hughes J, Mohs R, Heyman A. Detection of abnormal memory decline in mild cases of Alzheimer's disease using CERAD neuropsychological measures. Arch Neurol 1991;48:278–81.

46. Corder EH, Saunders AM, Strittmatter WJ, et al. Gene dose of apolipoprotein E type 4 allele and the risk of Alzheimer's disease in late onset families. Science 1993;261:921–3.

47. Strittmatter WJ, Saunders AM, Schmechel D, et al. Apolipoprotein E: high-avidity binding to beta-amyloid and increased frequency of type 4 allele in late-onset familial Alzheimer disease. Proc Natl Acad Sci USA 1993;90:1977–81.

48. Saunders AM, Strittmatter WJ, Schmechel D, et al. Association of apolipoprotein E allele epsilon 4 with late-onset familial and sporadic Alzheimer's disease. Neurology 1993;43:1467–72.

49. Mayeux R, Stern Y, Ottman R, et al. The apolipoprotein epsilon 4 allele in patients with Alzheimer's disease. Ann Neurol 1993;34:752–4.

50. Petersen RC, Smith GE, Ivnik RJ, et al. Apolipoprotein E status as a predictor of the development of Alzheimer's disease in memory-impaired individuals [published erratum appears in JAMA 1995;274:538]. JAMA 1995;273:1274–8.

51. Tierney MC, Szalai JP, Snow WG, et al. A prospective study of the clinical utility of ApoE genotype in the prediction of outcome in patients with memory impairment. Neurology 1996;46:149–54.

52. Poirier J, Delisle MC, Quirion R, et al. Apolipoprotein E4 allele as a predictor of cholinergic deficits and treatment outcome in Alzheimer disease. Proc Natl Acad Sci USA 1995;92:12260–4.

53. McBee WL, Dailey ME, Dugan E, Shumaker SA. Hormone replacement therapy and other potential treatments for dementias. Endocrinol Metab Clin North Am 1997;26:329–45.

54. Teng EL, Chui HC. The modified mini-mental state (3MS) examination. J Clin Psychiatry 1987;48:314–18.

55. Schneider LS, Farlow MR, Henderson VW, Pogoda JM. Effects of estrogen replacement therapy on response to tacrine in patients with Alzheimer's disease. Neurology 1996;46:1580–4.

56. Farlow MR, Lahiri DK, Poirier J, Davignon J, Hui S. Apolipoprotein E genotype and gender influence response to tacrine therapy. Ann NY Acad Sci 1996;802:101–10.

57. Knopman D, Schneider L, Davis K, et al. Long-term tacrine (Cognex) treatment: effects on nursing home placement and mortality, Tacrine Study Group. Neurology 1996;47:166–77.

58. Molnar FJ, Dalziel WB. The pharmacoeconomics of dementia therapies. Bringing the clinical, research and economic perspectives together. Drugs Aging 1997;10:219–33.

Regulatory issues in anti-dementia drug development

Peter J Whitehouse

5

The epidemiologic challenge of dementia is enormous and results in considerable personal and social stress (see chapters 9 and 10). The development of more effective medications to treat Alzheimer's disease (AD) and other dementia is a goal for many national and international groups. In this chapter we will review how decisions are made in different countries about which drugs should be granted regulatory approval. In most discussions of anti-dementia drug development, great emphasis is placed on basic biology and clinical studies, but it is actually these regulatory processes that reflect society's values about what therapeutic goals are desirable and what risks are acceptable.

We will first review draft or completed guidelines of a variety of national or regional bodies, including the Food and Drug Administration (FDA) in the USA, the European Medicines Evaluation Agency (EMEA) in Europe, the published unofficial Canadian Guidelines, and the guidelines that are being developed in Japan and China. Next, we will move to a consideration of the International Conference on Harmonization (ICH), a group that is attempting to standardize the process of submitting a global dossier to support a new drug application. We will than review the activities of the International Working Group on Harmonization of Dementia Drug (IWG), which is focusing on international drug studies of dementia. Finally, we will draw some conclusions about the regulatory environment that is likely to exist in the future.

National and regional regulatory guidelines

USA

Guidelines for the clinical evaluation of anti-dementia drugs were prepared by Dr Paul Leber, Director of the FDA's Division of Neuropharmacological Drug Products and were published in draft form on 8 November 1990.[1] The guidelines are divided into seven sections and focus principally on the phase II and phase III development of drugs to treat cognitive symptoms of AD. The guidelines were developed to assist sponsors in planning, designing, conducting and interpreting clinical investigations. Although they focus on

AD, they provide general principles relevant to other dementia. The core symptoms of intellectual impairment and ability to learn are said to be the targets of unmodified anti-dementia claims. The concept of pseudospecificity is discussed in an important footnote (p. 6, no. 3). Pseudospecificity is said to occur when a sponsor studies a new drug only in dementia, e.g. to treat depression, yet claims a dementia-specific action of the drug. Until recently, this statement about pseudospecificity contributed to a challenging environment for studies of how drugs affect the behavioral symptoms of dementia. It is important to recognize both the issues surrounding pseudospecific claims and the importance of developing more effective therapies for those non-cognitive aspects.

The FDA document includes considerable basic information about the purpose of clinical trials through all three phases of development. A preference for placebo as an internal control is asserted, although other approaches are said to be permissible under appropriate conditions, including the use of subtherapeutic doses of other drugs. A preference for parallel rather than cross-over studies is asserted.

The assessment of efficacy requires two primary outcome variables: a global assessment performed by a skilled clinician and a performance-based objective assessment of cognitive functions. Two types of global assessment are discussed, including global assessment of change and overall assessment of severity. Relatively little attention is paid to measuring clinical impact based on activities of daily living (ADLs), as, for example, with caregiver ratings.

Supplemental information is also provided by the FDA, including the appropriate use of data sets and imputation schemes. This supplement provides some more specific guidance about different forms of analysis.

Additional material is included in a letter addressed to potential sponsors concerning problems with the clinical global assessment, which were discovered by the FDA division as a consequence of analyzing submitted protocols. This letter identifies the need for the clinical global impression to be conducted independently of the objective psychometric test. Thus, the clinician conducting the global assessment should not have access to any results of the neuropsychometric tests, because they might bias the interpretation of the clinical global assessment.

In the letter, the Clinician Interview Based Impression of Change (CIBIC) is proposed as a model instrument. The CIBIC is to be given the same degree of weight in assessment of medications as the clinical global assessment proposed in the original anti-dementia drug guidelines. An essential feature of the CIBIC continues to be its independence from psychometric assessment. The CIBIC was originally proposed to be based entirely on information collected from the patient, so as not to be colored by any unblinding or other factors that might occur in a caregiver interview. The letter also discusses the possibility of using ADL assessments as a measure of clinical meaningfulness.

In subsequent meetings of the Peripheral and Central Nervous Science System Committee of the FDA, the concept of the CIBIC Plus was proposed by this author and others. The CIBIC Plus would allow an interview with the caregiver to be included in the performance of the CIBIC. (Perhaps in retrospect the use of the 'plus' modification seems a little nonsensical linguistically, but it indicates the addition of the caregiver as a source of information.) Moreover, ADL scales were given additional credence at these hearings, although with both the CIBIC Plus and

ADL assessments, the appropriate concern was raised that caregivers might be unblinded or influenced by other factors. During these meetings a motion proposed by this author was passed unanimously by the committee, to develop guidelines for drugs to treat non-cognitive and behavioral symptoms, such guidelines may evolve from international collaborative efforts described later.

It is important to emphasize the openness of the process that the FDA conducted. The initial draft guidelines were circulated widely, and input was provided from industry, academics, and other interested parties. Hearings were held in which the guidelines were discussed and modifications were made to the original positions of the agency. At the same time, new drug applications were submitted. After three hearings, tacrine was approved in 1993. Thus, the approval of the first drug in AD was the result of an interaction between the guidelines, the data submitted by the sponsor, and public meetings. However, officially the FDA guidelines continue to have draft status.

Europe

In Europe there has been a similarly long process of developing guidelines for the approval of AD medications. The EMEA guidelines[2] went through over a dozen versions and were finally approved in July 1997, making them the only official guidelines in modern times. They became operational in January 1998.

According to the EMEA, discussion began in the efficacy working party of the Committee for Proprietary Medicinal Products (CPMP) in October 1992. The process in Europe involved work by this committee as well as by the EMEA. This later agency came into effect officially in London on 1 January 1995. Hence, the process of developing guidelines in Europe involved a dynamic process, with the CPMP reflecting the old confederation of interested national bodies working in Europe and a new centralized body representing the new European Union. The draft FDA guidelines also influenced the European process. Currently, companies can elect to submit new drug applications centrally (as was done for propentofylline) or through individual countries (as was done for donepezil in the UK). Each path has different mechanisms with advantages and disadvantages. Both can lead to pan-European approval.

As with the FDA guidelines, the EMEA guidelines were transmitted on several occasions to interested parties. This author recalls commenting on three different occasions throughout the history of these guidelines. Unlike the FDA, the CPMP had to deal with considerable individual differences between countries, such as the UK, France, Germany, the Netherlands, and others.

Although earlier versions referred to multi-infarct dementia as well as AD, the final guidelines focus only on the treatment of AD. There is some recognition in this document, just as in the FDA document, that the guidelines may be adapted for use in other forms of dementia. There is also recognition that instrumentation for the assessment of some outcomes, such as ADLs and behavioral symptoms, is not yet at the same stage as instrumentation for assessment of cognitive symptoms. As in the FDA guidelines, the diagnosis of AD refers to the criteria of the NINDS-ADRDA (National Institute of Neurological Disorders and Stroke/Alzheimer Disease and Related Disorders Association).[3] Specific mention is made also of the 1993 criteria of the NINDS-AIREN (National Institute of Neurological Disorders and Stroke/Association Internationale

pour la Recherche et l'Enseignement en Neurosciences)[4] to exclude vascular dementia.

The document is divided into several sections: diagnosis, assessment of therapeutic efficacy, and general strategy. It is considerably briefer than the FDA document.

There are differences between the EMEA guidelines and the FDA document in the area of assessment of therapeutic efficacy. The European document points out that there are other goals besides symptomatic improvement (e.g. prevention or slowing progression), although the document focuses principally on symptomatic improvements. The guidelines suggest that cognitive symptoms should be assessed by objective psychometric tests and tests of ADL as well as by overall clinical response as reflected in global assessment. Hence, they add a third assessment area to the two included by the FDA, namely the assessment of ADL.

The EMEA guidelines also ask for a responder analysis. The definition of responders is left open, but the document suggests that there must be a prespecified degree of improvement in one cognitive end-point, with lack of worsening in the two other domains. The guidelines specifically mention that the end-points of interest may include behavioral symptoms, but highlights the importance of specifically focusing on those symptoms as a target. The document also suggests that changes in cognitive performance may be less important in more severely demented patients.

The EMEA document echoes the FDA recommendation that assessment in each domain should be done by a different investigator, to avoid contaminating assessments in the three areas. The characteristics of these areas (objective psychometric tests, tests of self-care and ADL, and global assessments) are included.

The document refers to two types of clinical assessment: global assessment and comprehensive assessment. The global scale is said to be single subjective integrated judgment, whereas comprehensive assessment may be a composite score of several domains. The CIBIC is identified as one example of global assessment, whereas the Clinical Dementia Rating is mentioned as one form of comprehensive assessment. Specific mention is made of

quality of life as an important dimension of assessment, but one requiring further work in instrumentation.[6]

The EMEA document concludes with some comments about general strategies in phases I, II and III which do not differ much from those in the FDA guidelines. There is specific mention that clinical trials should last for 6 months. However, studies of 1 year or more are considered desirable to evaluate the maintenance of efficacy. Further, 12-month studies are recommended for demonstrating long-term safety. In general, the EMEA guidelines recommend longer trial period than the FDA guidelines.

The EMEA guidelines also reflect an interest in defining subgroups of patients with AD. The document lists a variety of specific prognostic factors, such as apolipoprotein E genotype, severity of dementia, and presence of vascular risk factors, as possible modifiers of therapeutic response.

In conclusion, the European guidelines are briefer and reflect some recent research trends, such as interest in predicting therapeutic responsiveness and assessing quality of life. They differ from the FDA guidelines mainly in recommending longer trial periods and the use of three primary outcome measures. Moreover, they raise the question of responder analysis but provide little detail about how this should be conducted.

Canada

The Canadian guidelines were published in 1995.[7] The authors were leaders of the Consortium of Canadian Centers for Clinical Cognitive Research (C5R). The guidelines were developed with input from regulators from the Canadian government but are unofficial. Attempts have been made to see if Canada will develop official guidelines, but so far that decision has not been made.

The Canadian guidelines are notable for their comprehensiveness. They include major sections on diagnosis and therapeutic design, including considerable discussion of the different phases of studies. They devote considerable attention to measurement, including fairly extensive discussion of behavioral domains and ADL. In addition, more attention is paid than in other guidelines to the possible use of structural and functional imaging. Finally, the guidelines mention attempts to stabilize or slow progression of disease.

The report makes several specific recommendations, such as that research diagnostic criteria should be developed for all major causes of degenerative dementia, and that therapeutic goals should be defined broadly to include all disease stages. Thus, these guidelines are notable in making reference to other dementias and to the different stages of severity of AD. The document also recognizes the need for developing additional scales, particularly in the area of behavior and ADL. There is also brief discussion of the important issue of measuring pharmacoeconomic impact. Regarding assessment of cognition, these authors argue that approval for symptomatic treatment should require demonstration of efficacy within at least one of the individual domains of cognition, behavior, or function. In this suggestion the report differs from the FDA and EMEA guidelines. In discussing claims for stabilization of disease course, the authors point out that global staging is more appropriate for outcome assessment but that the distinction between long-term symptomatic effects and stabilization of course need to be clarified.

The Canadian document is rich in discussion of new potential scientific approaches, including neuroimaging and molecular biology (as might be expected from unofficial academic guidelines). Although supported with input from the Health Protection Branch and some other government agencies, this is an academic review of therapeutic opportunities in dementia. It has been influential in fostering discussion of therapeutic trial design not only in Canada but also in other countries.

Japan

The efforts of the Japanese governments to develop guidelines for the treatment of dementia include both the oldest guidelines and the newest. The old guidelines[8] were written at a time when such drugs were available on the clinical market. The document included discussion of the different phases of clinical developments, including phases I, II and III. What is important to recognize is that these were general guidelines for trials of both acute and chronic cerebral vascular disease. Thus, these guidelines were designed to be relevant to any situation in which cognitive impairment had occurred as a result of stroke. The guidelines include

discussions of accuracy of diagnosis, use of appropriate controls, identification of therapeutic goals, and attention to human rights, including placing a first priority on safety. Such emphasis on safety seems characteristic of the Japanese approach, but we must recognize that no efficacy standards existed in the USA until 1962. Patients with cerebral hemorrhage, cerebral infarction, transient ischemic attack and subarachnoid hemorrhages were included. Outcome measures felt to be necessary included general physical findings, subjective symptoms, psychiatric signs, neurologic signs, and ADL. Relatively little specification was given as to how improvement should be assessed in those areas, however.

A discussion of phase IV clinical trials was also included, because in Japan there is a system of post-approval reexamination of the drug. In fact, at the moment the Japanese Ministry of Health and Welfare is asking companies that had drugs approved on the basis of these old guidelines to submit new data to demonstrate efficacy. A considerable number of cerebral metabolic enhancers were approved in Japan, starting with the reference compound calcium hopatanate. Well-controlled studies were not conducted as a rule, and many drugs were approved on the basis of showing comparable efficacy with the difference compound rather than with placebo. As a result of this process, many cerebral metabolic enhancers appeared on the Japanese market with standards for efficacy that would not meet scrutiny today.

The Japanese Ministry of Health and Welfare announced in 1995 that it would develop guidelines for both vascular dementia and AD. The vascular dementia guidelines would be written as part of a review of the general guidelines for the development of medications to treat vascular disease. These vascular guidelines have been difficult to rewrite because multiple cerebral metabolic enhancers are available for the treatment of vascular disease, including dementia. The AD guidelines were influenced by the discussions that have occurred in the International Working Group on Harmonization of Dementia Drug Guidelines (see below in the International Guidelines). We expect that the Japanese guidelines will be completed in early 1998, but that there will then be a process of approval by the government (Homma and Sawada, personal communication).

Thus, the Japanese guidelines are notable for explicitly including vascular dementia and for being the latest guidelines to be developed, and thus influenced by international harmonization activities.

International Conference on Harmonization

The ICH comprises a group of regulators, principally from the USA, Japan, and Europe, with observers from other countries, notably Canada. The express purpose of this group is to improve and stardardize the process by which new drug applications are submitted in member countries. The secretariat for the ICH is the International Federation of Pharmaceutical Manufacturers' Association. The principal participants have thereby been regulators and scientists from industry, and there has been input from academics.

The first ICH conference was held in Brussels in 1991.[9] Additional conferences were held in Orlando, Florida,[10] in Yokohama, Japan, and most recently in 1996 in Brussels. One dissemination mechanism is an annual conference book. Examination of these books reveals particular discussion of the process by which data are collected and submitted for regulatory consideration. Thus, attention is being paid not only to the clinical development of a drug but also to the submission of preclinical data. The aim to try to standardize as much as possible both the content of the global dossier and its structure and process of submission. Notably, this group has not paid particular attention to specific diseases, although this may change in the future. One of relevance to studies in dementia is a special report on issues relating to drug studies in geriatric patients.

The ICH process has gone slowly because of the differences in existing regulatory structures and the politics of working towards global harmonization. Originally, three meetings were to be scheduled, but now a fourth has occurred, and perhaps others will be added. Apparently there is some interest in the group about examining disease-specific issues, but as for now no such attempts have been made. This process is important, however, because it provides the conceptual umbrella under which other groups may work to develop more harmonized approaches to drug development in specific disease categories.

International Working Group on Harmonization of Dementia Drug Guidelines

The IWG is one such group that is following in the footsteps of the ICH, focusing its attention exclusively on drugs for dementia.[11] This group was formed at the suggestion of the author and had its first meeting at the International Alzheimer's Conference in Minneapolis in July 1994. Dr Paul Leber from the FDA attended this preliminary meeting of approximately 50 academics and industry scientists. This group determined that there would be value in having an organization that would attempt to examine the draft guidelines from Canada, the USA and Europe. The overall goal is greater efficiency in multinational multisite studies so that better drugs can be developed less expensively.

After the initial meeting in Minneapolis, a survey was taken of interested participants and a number of committees were established (Table 5.1). Committees were divided into major blocks: those dealing with outcome measurements, such as objective psychometric tests, global assessment, ADL, and quality of life; those dealing with design issues around trials for

Table 5.1
Committees of the International Working Group on Harmonization of Dementia Drug Guidelines: Working Group/Facilitators.

ADL

Dr Serge Gauthier, McGill Centre for Studies in Aging, Douglas Hospital, 6825 LaSalle Boulevard, Verdun (Quebec), Canada H4H 1R3

Tel: 514-766-2010/Fax: 514-888-4050

E-mail: mcmu@musica.mcgill.ca

Clinical global measures

Dr Barry Reisberg, Clinical Director, Aging & Dementia Research Center, Millhauser Labs (HN-314), N.Y.U. Medical Center, 550 First Avenue, New York, NY 10016, USA

Tel: 212-263-5700/Fax: 212-263-6991

E-mail: barry.reisberg@mcadr.med.nyu.edu

Cultural issues

Dr Luigi A. Amaducci, University of Florence, Department of Neurology & Psychiatry Science, Viale Morgagni 85, Florence, Italy

Tel: (39)55.43.2224/Fax: (39)55.41.3603

E-mail: pfinv@server.area.fi.cnr.it

Diagnostic criteria

Dr Zaven Khachaturian, Director, Reagan Research Institute, 8912 Copenhaver Drive, Potomac, MD 20854, USA

Tel: 301-879-2582/Fax: 301-217-0054

E-mail: zaven@haven.ios.com

Ethical issues

Dr Stephen Post, Associate Professor, Biomedical Ethics, Philosophy, and Religion, Case Western Reserve University, Center for Biomedical Ethics, 10900 Euclid Avenue, SCM, Cleveland, OH 44106-4976,USA

Tel: 216-368-6205/Fax: 216-368-8713

E-mail: sgp2@po.cwru.edu

Information systems

Dr Richard Harvey, Dementia Research Group, The National Hospital for Neurology and Neurosurgery, Queen Square, London WC1N 3BG, UK

Tel: (4417)-18373611/Fax: (4417)-12090182

E-mail: r.harvey@ic.ac.uk

Table 5.1 *continued*
Committees of the International Working Group on Harmonization of Dementia Drug Guidelines: Working Group/Facilitators.

Objective psychometric tests

Dr Steven Ferris, Director, Alzheimer's Disease Center, New York University School of Medicine, Aging and Dementia Research Center, Room THN 312B, 550 First Avenue, New York, NY 10016, USA

Tel: 212-263-5703/Fax: 212-263-6991

E-mail: steven.ferris@mcadr.med.nyu.edu

Pharmacoeconomics

Dr Bengt Winblad, Department of Clinical Neuroscience and Family Medicine, Karolinska Institutet, Huddinge University Hospital, Division of Geriatric Medicine, B84, S-141 86, Huddinge, Sweden

Tel: 46-858-585474/Fax: 46-858-58570

E-mail: bengt.winblad@cnsf.ki.se

Prevention protocols

Dr Leon Thal, Department of Neurosciences, University of California, 9500 Gilman Drive, LaJolla, CA 92023, USA

Tel: 619-534-4606/Fax: 619-534-1437

E-mail: Lthal@ucsd.edu

Protocols to demonstrate slowing progression of disease

Dr Martin Rossor, The National Hospital for Neurology & Neurosurgery, Queen Square, London WC1N 2BG, UK

Tel: (4417)-18373611/Fax: (4417)-12090182

E-mail: m.rossor@ic.ac.uk

Protocols for treating non-cognitive symptoms

Dr Akira Homma, Tokyo Metropolitan Institute of Gerontology, Department of Psychiatry, 35-2 Sakae-cho, Itabashi-ku, Tokyo 173, Japan

Tel: (81)338-643241/Fax: (81)335-794776

E-mail: ahomma@tmig.or.jp

Quality of life

Dr Peter Whitehouse, Professor of Neurology, University Alzheimer Center, 12200 Fairhill Road, C323, Cleveland, OH 44120, USA

Tel: 216-844-7361/Fax: 216-844-6369

E-mail: pjw3@po.cwru.edu

Dr Jean-Marc Orgogozo, Université de Bordeaux, Département de Neurologie, Hôpital Pellegrin, 33076 Bordeaux Cedex, France
Tel: 3-35.56.79.6004/Fax: 3-35.56.98.1378
E-mail: i.m.orgogozo@neuro.u-bordeaux2.fr

Translation
Dr Howard Feldman, University Hospital Division of Neurology, Vancouver Hospital & Health Sciences Center, S192-2211 Wesbrook Mall, Vancouver BC, Canada V6T 2B5
Tel: 604-822-7697/Fax: 604-822-7703
E-mail: hfeldman@unixg.ubc.ca

Dr Luis Fornazzari, Neurology-Neuropsychiatry Research, Universidad de Chile, Departamento Salud Mental Area Oriente, Instituto Psiquiatrico, Alvaro Casanova 1941, La Reina Santiago, Chile
Tel: 56-227-39294/Fax: 56-227-39294
E-mail: Forna@mali.mic.cl

Vascular dementia
Dr Timo Erkinjuntti, Chief, Memory Research Unit, Helsinki University Central Hospital, Department of Clinical Neurosciences, Haartmaninkatu 4, FIN-00290 Helsinki, Finland
Tel: 3-589-4712353/Fax: 3-589-4712352
E-mail: timo.erkinjuntti@HUCH.FI

Dr Tohru Sawada, Executive Director, BF Research Institute, c/o National Cardiovascular Center, 5-7-1 Fujishirodai, Suita-shi, Osaka 565, Japan
Tel: (81)683-47646/Fax: (81)687-28761
E-mail: sawadato@po.iijnet.or.jp

South American regional
Dr Carlos Mangone, Assistant Professor of Neurology, University of Buenos Aires, Hospital Municipal D. Francisco Santojanni, Servicio de Neurologia, Pilar 950, 1480 Buenos Aires, Argentina
Tel: 541-982-6259/Fax: 541-961-5715
E-mail: cmangone@logos.com.ar

European regional
Dr Jean-Marc Orgogozo, Université de Bordeaux, Département de Neurologie, Hôpital Pellegrin, 33076 Bordeaux Cedex, France
Tel: 3-35.56.79.6004/Fax: 3-35.56.98.1378
E-mail: j.m.orgogozo@neuro.u-bordeaux2.fr

behavioral symptoms, slowing the progression of disease, and prevention; and those dealing with broader issues that affect drug development, including translation, cultural differences, and ethical issues. Each committee was charged with reviewing the draft guidelines, examining what differences existed, and specifying a program of research. The committees worked electronically, by fax and e-mail, to produce draft documents that were based on literature searches and expert opinion. These documents were presented at a meeting held at the Royal Society of Medicine in September 1995. The final reports were published in 1997.[11]

The IWG meets on a regular basis at the International Alzheimer's Conference and last met as a whole in Osaka, Japan in July 1996. The focus of the Osaka meeting was on the draft European guidelines that became official the following year.

The IWG has found it particularly important to work alongside other international organizations with similar interests in improving the efficiency of anti-dementia drug development. Associated organizations include: the World Federation of Neurology Research Section on Dementia; the International Psychogeriatric Association; Alzheimer Disease International; the confederation of national family organizations; the International Pharmaceutical Manufacturers' Association, to provide connection to the ICH; and the World Health Organization, which has officially recognized the meetings of the IWG.

The strategy adopted by the IWG in the future will be to develop meetings on topics of particular interest to its members and the field, in addition to its regular meetings every two years. Thus, several regional meetings have been held in Japan (1996), Canada (1996), China (1997), and Europe (1997). Topics focusing on specific content areas have also been developed. A meeting was held with Alzheimer's Disease International in Helsinki in 1997 on the important topic of informed consent in research. This process will lead to publication of a consensus document in *Alzheimer's Disease and Associated Disorders*. A conference on pharmacoeconomics is planned for July 1998 in Amsterdam and a conference on vascular dementia will be held in October 1998 in Osaka. Other areas of planning include conferences in slowing progression of disease, behavioral symptoms, and quality of life.

The IWG is expanding its activities to include countries and regions of the world that are not part of the ICH process. Active collaborations have been established in China, both to help facilitate multicenter drug trials and to work with the Chinese government on the development of guidelines. In South America, active efforts are ongoing in Argentina, Chile and Uruguay to develop multicenter studies and to work with governments to enhance the visibility of AD as a public policy concern. A South American Regional Committee has been recently established.

Conclusions and future trends

The development of anti-dementia drugs will probably continue to be a major priority of patients and families, clinicians, the pharmaceutical industry, and governments. Nevertheless, a number of areas of change are likely to dramatically affect the process in the future, ranging from basic biological science to public policy and ethics.

New discoveries in basic biology, particularly the discovery of new genetic abnormalities that cause AD and related disorders, will continue to fuel the pipeline of ideas for new drugs. We seem to be moving beyond symptomatic treatments based on neurotransmitter system abnormalities to interventions that may slow the progression of disease by slowing the death of nerve cells or the formation of pathologic features, particularly amyloid deposition. These basic science discoveries will be combined with a variety of new preclinical pharmaceutical industry techniques, ranging from genomics to combinational chemistry and high-throughput screening. Thus, more candidates are likely to arrive for clinical evaluation over the next decades.

However, there will be many complex challenges around the issue of conducting clinical trials. There are well-accepted trial designs for studying drugs that treat cognitive symptoms, but there are still major issues in designing trials to demonstrate that a drug improves behavior, slows progression, or prevents the disease.

Regardless of the nature of the design for a particular protocol, there will continue to be major attempts to improve the efficiency of clinical trials.

In addition, there will be continued attempts to reconsider the traditional approach of drug development in four phases. Perhaps efficacy measures should be introduced earlier in drug development to see if clues to dosage can be obtained. Moreover, it is likely that data that have traditionally been collected in phase IV, namely, quality of life and cost data, will be incorporated into earlier phases of drug evaluation.

Academic centers in the USA and probably in other countries will face increasing competitive pressure to conduct research in more efficient ways. For-profit companies have been established that may be able to provide higher-quality data than those traditionally obtained from academic centers. Clinical research organizations and other groups were formed in an attempt to develop the necessary clinical data for regulatory approval in new and more effective ways.[12]

Although randomized controlled studies should remain the gold standard, we may have to consider what other sources of data could be used to help us make decisions about the use of particular medications. Other forms of evidence, be it epidemiologic data or systematic clinical observations, may have to fit into our decision-making process in different ways than currently.[13,14]

The promise is great that future drugs will have more fundamental impacts on the disease. However, the simple claim that these drugs will save money needs to be examined carefully. Thus, the whole area of pharmacoeconomics in dementia is likely to become more important. Pharmacoeconomics is a relatively new science, and relatively little attention has been paid to chronic diseases such as AD. Such studies will be increasingly important, as it appears that getting regulatory approval for a drug is becoming almost secondary to the process of getting a drug evaluated and paid for by a healthcare system. Pharmacoeconomic studies will also raise the important issue of assessment of quality of life, an area that until recently has been relatively neglected in studies of dementia.[6] Payers will be looking for a more profound impact on disease than merely an effect on an objective psychometric test or on a clinician's impression of change.

The regulatory agencies that represent one of the forms of social control on the development of new drugs are also undergoing rapid change. In the near future, certain changes may occur in the manner that drugs are evaluated. For example, there has been increasing attention given to the question of whether two studies are necessary or whether one carefully designed study would be adequate for the approval of a drug. The EMEA is still young. There is an evolution in its responsibilities in relation to the Committee for Proprietary Medicinal Products which, until the formation of the EMEA, had sole responsibility for pan-European activities. In Japan, major scandals due to products contaminated by HIV have limited the activities of the Ministry of Health and Welfare. In general, however, Japanese leaders seem to be interested in developing guidelines that will meet international standards. Drug evaluation in less industrialized countries is also evolving rapidly, particularly driven by the aging of their populations.

The Chinese population is aging very rapidly, and major social upheavals are likely in the early part of the next century as a result of the imbalance between the number of individuals in the workforce and the number of retired individuals. China also offers us an opportunity to systematically examine other forms of medical treatment for dementia. In China, Western medicines are actually an alternative approach to treating dementia, and a variety of traditional techniques, including herbs and acupuncture, will continue to be used. In the USA and other industrial countries, interest is growing in these complementary approaches. The social roots of this interest may prove challenging to pharmaceutical companies as they try to compete with these products for patients' resources.[15-18]

Anti-dementia drug development will also be increasingly affected by reconsideration of ethical issues. We need to be sensitive to both universal and local ethical principles concerning the conduct of drug trials. Some major issues remain unresolved, including how to assess competence to consent, how to identify surrogates, and how to assess the relative risks and benefits of a protocol for a patient with dementia.

The future of drug development in AD looks bright from a biological perspective, at least for modest gains, but drug development will occur in an increasingly complex political and healthcare environment, that will surely affect the process as much as our discoveries in basic biology.

References

1. Leber P. Guidelines for clinical evaluation of antidementia drugs. Washington, DC: US Food and Drug Administration, 1990.

2. CPMP Working Party on Efficacy of Medicinal Products. Note for Guidance. (The European Agency for the Evaluation of Medicinal Products Human Medicines Evaluation Unit: London, 1997).

3. McKann G, Arachman D, Folstein M, et al. Clinical diagnosis of Alzheimer's disease: Report of the NINCDS-ADRDA work group. Neurology 1984;34:939-44.

4. Roman GC, Tatemichi TK, Erkinjuntti T, et al. Vascular dementia: diagnostic criteria for research studies. Report of the NINDS-AIREN international work group. Neurology 1993;43:250-60.

5. Morris JC. The Clinical Dementia Rating (CDR): current version and scoring rules. Neurology 1993; 43:2412-14.

6. Whitehouse PJ. Quality of life in dementia. In: Winbald B, Wimo A, Jonsson B, Karlsson G, eds. Health economics of dementia. Chichester: John Wiley & Sons, in press.

7. Mohr E, Feldman H, Gauthier S. Canadian guidelines for the development of antidementia therapies: a conceptual summary. Can J Neurol Sci 1995;22:62-71.

8. Study Team for Establishment of Clinical Evaluation Procedures for Cerebral Circulation and Metabolism Improvers. Guideline on Clinical Evaluation of Cerebral Circulation and Metabolism Improvers. (Study Team for Establishment of Clinical Evaluation Procedures for Cerebral Circulation and Metabolism Improvers: Tokyo, 1986).

9. D'Arcy PF, Harron DWG, eds. Proceedings of the First International Conference on Harmonization, Orlando, Florida, 1991; Belfast: Queen's University, 1991.

10. D'Arcy PF, Harron DWG, eds. Proceedings of the Second International Conference on Harmonization, Orlando, Florida, 1993; Belfast: Queen's University, 1993.

11. Report of the International Working Group on Harmonization of Dementia Drug Guidelines. Alzheimer Disease Assoc Disord 1997;11(suppl 3):1-64.

12. Industry Review Report. Academic medical centers: slowly turning the tide. Center Watch Inc 1997;4:6:1-8.

13. Jonas WB. Clinical trials for chronic disease. J NIH Res 1997;9:33-9.

14. Pincus T. Controversies in science. J NIH Res 1997;9:32-8.

15. Sun Y, Whitehouse PJ. Traditional Chinese medicine therapeutic approaches to dementia. In preparation.

16. Zhibao X, Xuelan S, eds. A Guide of the Treatment by Traditional Chinese Medicine (Dongzhimen Hospital Beijing University of Traditional Chinese Medicine: Beijing, 1995).

17. Fan WJ-W. A manual of Chinese herbal medicine. Principles and practice for easy reference. Boston: Shambhala Publications, 1996.

18. Ikels C. The experience of dementia in China. Culture Med Psychiatry (in press).

Cholinesterase inhibitors for Alzheimer's disease therapy: Pharmacokinetic and pharmacodynamic considerations

Ezio Giacobini

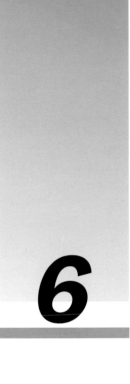

6

Development of cholinesterase inhibitors for Alzheimer's disease therapy: from tacrine to second generation

Cholinergic deficits in Alzheimer's disease (AD) have been well documented.[1] The reductions in cortical and cerebrospinal fluid (CSF) cholinergic markers are correlated with the extent of the neuropathology and with the severity of cognitive impairment. We assume that low concentrations (nM) of acetylcholine (ACh) in cortical synapses would severely impair its neuromodulatory effects on non-cholinergic neurons.

We calculated that the difference in cortical ACh levels between normal elderly controls and AD patients is of the order of 50%.[2] We can therefore postulate that a cholinesterase inhibitor (ChEI) capable of doubling ACh levels from approximately 150 nM to 300 nM would re-establish a close-to-normal level of neurotransmitter. All ChEIs tested in the author's laboratory with intracortical microdialysis have shown this capability.[3] Theoretically, they should also be able to produce cognitive improvement in AD patients. Experimental support for this hypothesis is provided by the results of Scali et al,[4] who demonstrated in aged rats a direct correlation between levels of AChE inhibition, increase in extracellular ACh levels in vivo in cortex and hippocampus, and cognitive improvement.[4]

The clinical application of ChEIs in the field of AD started in the early 1980s with the oral and intravenous administration of physostigmine.[5,6] The results of these first experimental treatments were encouraging, as they clearly demonstrated the potential of this pharmacological approach in reducing decline of cognitive function. However, the effect of physostigmine was too short in duration and the cholinergic side-effects too severe and frequent for the drug to be suitable for long-term treatment.

A historical breakthrough in the long-term treatment of AD with ChEIs occurred in the mid-1980s with the use of a different drug:[7] Summers et al reported the effect of oral administration of tetrahydroaminoacridine (tacrine, THA) for a period of 12.6 months in 17 patients. This study was preceded by a short-term pilot trial with the same drug administered intravenously to 12 AD patients.[8] It is interesting to note that tacrine was never intended to be a drug for the treatment of AD, and even less a ChEI.

Tacrine was first characterized pharmacologically by Shaw and Bentley[9] in Australia as an analeptic capable of causing rapid arousal of morphinized dogs and cats. Early clinical applications of tacrine were treatment of anaesthetic-induced delirium[10] and potentiation of the muscle-relaxing effect of succinylcholine.[11] In 1953, Shaw and Bentley[12] had shown that tacrine is almost as powerful a ChEI as eserine or neostigmine, producing 50% inhibition of ChE at concentrations of 10^{-7} M. However, it was not known whether or not the synergism of ChEI with succinylcholine depended upon a direct cholinergic effect or on inhibition of the enzymatic breakdown of the drug. Heilbronn[13] characterized for the first time the effect of tacrine upon acetylcholinesterase (AChE) and butyrylcholinesterase (BuChE). The clinical effect demonstrated by tacrine has substantiated this view.

Cholinesterase inhibitors: Do they work? Are there differences?

Cholinesterase inhibitors presently undergoing clinical trials in Japan, the USA and Europe include 10 drugs, most of which have already advanced to clinical phase III and IV, and three (tacrine, ENA 713 and donepezil) are registered in USA and/or in Europe.[3] It is likely that in the next 2-year period (1998–1999) at least three other ChEIs will be registered worldwide. Analysis of the results emerging from clinical trials poses two questions: are ChEIs efficacious in AD patients and, if so, how do these drugs work; and are there major differences among various compounds with regard to efficacy, percentage of treatable patients, dropouts and side-effects? These two fundamental questions can be partially answered by comparing recent clinical data (Table 6.1) emerging from studies using the same rating scales. Table 6.1 compares for the first time the effect of six ChEIs on the ADAS-Cog using ITT (intention-to-treat) criteria. The duration of these trials varied between 12 and 30 weeks and the total number of tested patients was above 6000. Based on the data reported in these studies, the answer to the first question is affirmative. All six ChEIs tested under similar criteria produce statistically significant improvements using a standardized and internationally validated measure of cognition. One first observation is the similarity in size of cognitive effect for all six drugs when expressed as a difference between drug- and placebo-treated patients. Differences in ADAS-Cog at all doses between drug- and placebo-treated patients average approximately 3.7 points (range 1.9–5.3). An average difference of 1.2 points is seen at the study end-point (range 0.5–2.8). This difference varies from 0.5 points (metrifonate high dose) to 2.8 points (tacrine high dose). As seen in Table 6.1, the difference in effect between low and high dose is not constantly dose dependent but seems to vary in relation to the therapeutic window of that particular drug. Similarity in cognitive effect size suggests a present ceiling value of approximately 5 ADAS-Cog points average for ChEI at mild to moderate stages of the disease (CDR 1–2). This may suggest that some drugs may not have been tested at their full capacity. Higher doses could still increase the effect size.

A similarity of clinical effect is also supported by the close values on global scales such as CIBIC-plus (Clinical Interview-based Impression of

Table 6.1
Comparison of the effect of six cholinesterase inhibitors on ADAS-Cog test (ITT)

Drug	Dose (mg./day)	Duration of study (weeks)	Treatment difference from Placebo*	Baseline**	Improved patients (%)	Dropout (%)	Side-effects (%)
Tacrine[15,16]	120–160	30	4.0–5.3	0.8–2.8	30–50	55–73	40–58
Eptastigmine[56,57]	45	25	4.7	1.8	30	12	35
Donepezil[17,64,65]	5–10	24	2.5–2.9	0.7–1	58	13–30	13
ENA 713[14]	6–12	24	1.9–4.9	0.7	25	15–27	28
Metrifonate[58–60]	25–75	12–26	2.8–3.1	0.75–0.5	35	2–21	2–12
Galanthamine[62]	30	12	3.3	1.8	–	33	–

ADAS-Cog, AD Assessment Scale–cognitive subscale; ITT, intention to treat; *study end-point versus placebo; **study end-point versus baseline; THA, tacrine.

Change-plus): an average of 0.4 points for tacrine, ENA 713 and metrifonate at 24 weeks. For tacrine, the high percentage of dropouts and side-effects seen suggests a practical limit of ChE inhibition as well as of drug effect. For other drugs (e.g. metrifonate and donepezil), in spite of a dosage producing high ChE inhibition (up to 80%), severity of side-effects does not seem to represent a limiting factor. In general, the percentage of improved patients varies from 25% (donepezil, high dose) to 50% (tacrine, high dose), with an average of 34%. This indicates that one-third of treated patients show a positive response (responders). Note that 20–25% of patients do not improve at all (non-responders). It is plausible to think that the percentage of treatable patients could be increased to 75–80% by using higher doses of those ChEIs which produce less severe side-effects. The available 6-month data suggest that patients treated with the active compound change little cognitively from baseline at the beginning of the trial to the end. As an example, in a US study with ENA 713, patients administered placebo for 26 weeks deteriorated by over 4 points on the ADAS-Cog

compared to only 0.3 in patients given 6–12 mg/day of the drug.[14]

The same trend is true for metrifonate-treated patients, who showed only a 0.5 point difference at week 26 of treatment. This may suggest that the difference between placebo-treated and drug-treated groups at 6 months may relate more to the rate of cognitive deterioration of the placebo group, which varies between 2 and 4 ADAS-cog points, than to a symptomatic effect of the drug. This putative protective effect could be primary and structural, leading to an improvement of cholinergic function as reflected by the cognitive improvement measured by ADAS-Cog, or be secondary. Tacrine and donepezil, on the other hand, seem to show a real initial symptomatic improvement (2–3 point gain) as compared to the placebo group. This effect may last from 4 to 24 weeks, depending on the dose.[15-17] It remains to be demonstrated whether or not this profile of improvement reflects a real difference in drug effect. As indicated by open-trial studies of longer duration (up to 24 months), it is possible to maintain the difference between placebo- and drug-treated subjects beyond the present 6-month limit for a period of 12 months or more. Thus, cholinesterase inhibitors may differ from one another with respect not only to magnitude but also to duration of effect.

In comparing results of different clinical trials and different drugs, one should take into consideration the fact that studies may differ one from another, depending on differences in selection criteria and age of subjects, severity of disease, concomitant illnesses, medications, instruments of assessment and side-effect evaluation. In addition to these variables, in order to evaluate differences in effect between drugs one has to take into consideration the rate of deterioration of the placebo-exposed group which is compared with the treatment group. The rate of deterioration seems to be highly variable (1–4 points on ADAC-Cog over 24 weeks) among different studies and populations of subjects. Thus, clinical studies are not entirely comparable with one another and conclusions need to be drawn with caution.

What makes the difference between various ChEIs? Pharmacokinetic and pharmacodynamic aspects

The relation between percentage peripheral (blood) ChE inhibition and

cognitive (ADAS-Cog) or global impression of change rated by the clinician (CGIC) effect is a relevant factor in understanding the mechanism of action. The data presented in Table 6.2 support the pharmacological concept that brain ChE inhibition leads to an improvement of functional ACh levels which benefits cognition. This relationship might vary quantitatively for each drug, so each compound may produce various levels of cognitive improvement and therapeutic effect.[2,3,18] This hypothesis is in agreement with pharmacological data in animals[19,20] and in humans.[18] The level of peripheral enzyme inhibition which has been measured in patients (AChE activity in erythrocytes or BuChE activity in plasma) correlating with cognitive effect varies between 30% and 80%, depending on kinetic and pharmacological characteristics of the compound (Table 6.2). For some drugs (donepezil and metrifonate) the achievable level of non-toxic ChE inhibition can be as high as 90%. As predicted by pharmacological and behavioural data, there is a clear correlation between ChE inhibition (or drug plasma concentration) and cognitive effect.[20,21] Drugs producing mild cholinergic side-effects at a high level of brain ChE inhibition have the advantage of being tested in the patient within their full range of therapeutic

Table 6.2
Relation between percentage cholinesterase inhibition and effect on ADAS-Cog or CGIC.

Drug	Dose mg/day	Steady state (% inhibition)	Optimal (% inhibition)	Correlation ChEl/ADAS-Cog or CGIC
Physostigmine[6]	3–16	40–60 (BuChE)	30–40	U-shaped
Eptastigmine[56,61]	30–60	13–54 (AChE)	30–35	U-shaped
Metrifonate[63]	30	35–75 (AChE)	65–80	U-shaped
Donepezil[64,65]	5	64 (AChE)	60	Linear
Tacrine[15,16]	160	40 (BuChE) 60 (AChE)	30	Linear
Galanthamine[62]	20–50	50–60 (AChE)	50	U-shaped

ADAS-Cog, AD Assessment Scale–cognitive subscale; CGIC, Clinician Global Impression of Change.

potential. For some ChEls (physostigmine, eptastigmine and metrifonate) the relation between ChE inhibition and cognitive effect is inversely-U shaped, while for other (e.g. tacrine, ENA 713 and donepezil) this relation seems to be linear. The U-shaped form can be explained by the fact that by increasing the dose of the inhibitor one obtains progressively increasing efficacy until adverse effects become a limiting factor. Thus, indirectly, the level of ChE inhibition may define the extent of the therapeutic window. A second reason for the U-shaped curve is the specific inhibition kinetic of the inhibitor- and the substrate-induced saturation effect of ChEs. The level of ACh brain elevation varies according to brain ChE inhibition.[2,3,22] With increased brain concentrations of ACh, substrate inhibition of enzyme activity becomes operational in vivo as it is observed in brain tissue in vitro.[22] Plotting the velocity of enzymatic reaction against substrate (ACh) concentration results in a bell-shaped curve with a defined peak in the case of AChE activity in brain and erythrocytes, and a sigmoid curve in the case of BuChE activity in plasma (Figure 6.1).[23] Thus, AChE activity is inhibited by a large excess of ACh, such as could be present following high inhibition of brain AChE in treated AD patients. Excessive elevation of the substrate has the effect of decreasing the catalytic

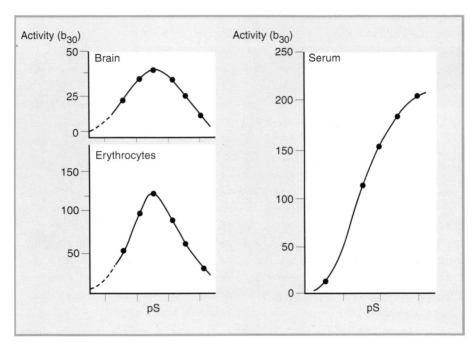

Figure 6.1
Effect of ACh concentration (pS) on the activity of AChE (Erythrocytes) and BuChE (Serum).

potency of the enzyme and subsequently its pharmacological and therapeutic effect. From this relationship it can be predicted that a high level of ChE inhibition reached rapidly during treatment will not further increase efficacy but only augment CNS-dependent side-effects (drowsiness, nausea, vomiting, etc). This concept is clearly illustrated by the example of oral physostigmine administration. It should

be an advantage to use a slow-release type of ChEI inhibiting both types of brain enzymes (AChE and BuChE) in order to reach slowly and gradually steady-state levels of brain ACh. This strategy may also lower the risk of cholinergic receptor downregulation and enzyme induction (see development of tolerance). It is known that central cholinergic side-effects which may develop early in the treatment may not be directly related to the level of brain AChE inhibition but rather to a rapid elevation of ACh levels.[2,22,24] Peripheral side-effects may occur which depend on a rapid redistribution of the drug (or its metabolites) between peripheral organs and muscles and the CNS. Because of the complex mechanism of action of ChEIs, reaching maximal clinical effect is more complicated than just elevating the dose at the maximal tolerated level. The last, but not the least, problem with ChEI therapy is the early identification of those patients most likely to benefit from therapy. Correlation of therapy effectiveness with genetic risk factors (such as the ApoE allele) represents a first but still controversial attempt in this direction. Choosing the proper responder to cholinomimetics and selecting patients at earlier stages of the disease may be crucial for the success of the therapy.

Long-term treatment and development of tolerance: a question of enzyme induction or of receptor regulation?

Tolerance to single or repeated doses of ChEI may contribute, together with patient deterioration, to progressively diminishing the clinical effect of the drug. There is a vast literature addressing the phenomenon of tolerance to both single and repeated doses of ChEI.[24-26] Adaptation to and decreased effect of ChEI are evident in behavioural as well as in toxicological studies.[27] Tolerance to repeated doses of ChEI might be explained by two mechanisms. The first is a reduction in sensitivity to ACh or a decreased number (downregulation) of muscarinic and nicotinic receptors. This explanation may be valid under experimental conditions but more difficult to apply to AD patients who suffer from a deficit in ACh synthesis and a decrease in nicotinic (not muscarinic) receptor number.

A second, more likely, explanation for tolerance may be an induced new synthesis of the AChE at nerve terminals which could be reflected by an increase level of AChE activity in CSF of treated AD patients. The AChE activity present in CSF originates from spinal cord and brain neurons as a result of a secretory process.[28,29] This secretion shows a tendency to decrease with severity of dementia and disease progression.[30]

Stimulation of AChE release from neurons into the CSF has been invoked by Bareggi and Giacobini[28] to explain increased AChE activity in the CSF of dogs after drug administration. An increase in CSF AChE activity in CSF was also found by Mattio et al[19] in dogs given high doses of physostigmine intraventricularly. These data relate CSF AChE activity to brain AChE activity. Several observations indicate that an increased production of both AChE and BuChE may occur in dogs and rats after long-term treatment with different ChEIs.[19,26]

Plasma BuChE activity, in particular, may overshoot the basal level for a time after dosing is stopped. Particularly relevant to clinical conditions is the increase in plasma BuChE activity seen in humans receiving chronic doses of organophosphates such as parathion orally or in spray form.[31,32] Plasma BuChE activity increased after 2–5 days of treatment and stabilized itself between day 7 and 10 of treatment. After the exposure was stopped, there was a rebound of ChE activity, sometimes reaching twice the normal level.[25,30] Is there a corresponding behavioural tolerance to ChEI? The answer seems to be affirmative. Behavioural adaptation to a number of ChEIs, from organophosphates to carbamates, has

been described in numerous publications.[26]

Reduction in sensitivity or in number (downregulation) of both muscarinic and nicotinic receptors after repeated doses of ChEI has been demonstrated to be associated with tolerance in several studies.[24-26] How can we cope with this problem in the clinic?

Two strategies which may avoid or limit tolerance to ChEI effects are the readjustment of the dose to higher levels during the course of treatment, or temporary discontinuation (wash-out periods) of treatment until AChE activity returns to baseline levels. This wash-out period is followed by a restart of treatment at the same or higher dose. A control of AChE activity in CSF relative to red blood cell AChE would be the most effective way to titrate dosage after long-term treatment with a ChEI. It is realized that such a strategy may not be easily implemented in the patient.

Should a cholinesterase inhibitor be selective for brain acetylcholinesterase?

The brain of mammals investigated so far, including humans, has been shown to contain two major forms of ChE, AChE and BuChE.[33] Using specific substrates and inhibitors, it has been shown that, in contrast to AChE, BuChE preferentially hydrolyses butyrylcholine.[34] Butyrylcholine is not a substrate in human brain.

By combination of specific substrates with selective inhibitors, it has been demonstrated that in rat brain approximately 80% activity is AChE and 20% is BuChE.[34] In rat brain, BuChE activity is mainly localized to glial cells, while AChE activity is mainly concentrated in nerve cells.[35,36] In the human brain, BuChE is found in both neurons and glia as well as in neuritic plaques and tangles in AD patients.[37]

Depending on the region, human brain AChE activity is 1.5-fold (temporal and parietal cortex) to 60-fold (caudate nucleus) higher than BuChE activity.[20,38-41]

An important feature distinguishing BuChE from AChE is its kinetics towards different concentrations of ACh. An excess of this substrate (μM) will inhibit AChE, but not BuChE. Because of the difference in K_m of the two enzymes, glial BuChE is less efficient in hydrolysing ACh at low

substrate concentrations (sub-micromolar) than neuronal AChE. What could be the consequence of this enzymatic kinetic difference?

The proportion of the two enzymes present in human brain is strongly altered in the course of AD. In the cortex of patients affected by AD, AChE activity decreases progressively to 10–15% of normal values, while BuChE activity is unchanged or even increased by 20%.[20,38-41] For example, the BuChE/AChE ratio will increase in AD from 0.6 to 0.9 in the frontal cortex and from 0.6 to 11 in the enthorinal cortex. This may be related to a combination of reactive gliosis and accumulation of BuChE in neuritic plaques.[37] It is likely that with a strongly decreased concentration of synaptic AChE, particularly the membrane-anchored G4 form, in the presence of a ChEI, ACh concentrations could reach micromolar levels which are inhibitory for AChE activity.[42,43] This increase may trigger glial BuChE to hydrolyse ACh in order to compensate for the loss of neuronal AChE activity. Due to the close anatomical and spatial relationships between glial cell protoplasm and the synaptic gap, it is likely that extracellularly diffusing ACh could come in contact

Table 6.3
In vitro activity (IC$_{50}$, nM) of cholinesterase inhibitors in human erythrocytes and plasma.[24]

Compound	AChE[a]	BuChE[b]	BuChE/AChE
BW 284 C51	18.8	48.000	2.553
Phenserine	22.2	1552	70
Galanthamine	0.35	18.6	53
DDVP (metrifonate)	800	18.000	22.5
Physostigmine	5.4	35	6.5
THA	190	47	0.25
Eptastigmine	20	5	0.25
Hetopropazine	260.000	300	0.001
Bambuterol	30.000	3	0.001
MF-8622	100.000	9	0.00009

[a]Human erythrocytes. [b]Human plasma.

with glial BuChE and be effectively hydrolysed, as demonstrated by experiments in the rat in vivo.[44]

To study the function of glial BuChE and in particular its effect on the regulation of ACh extracellular concentrations, rats were perfused intracortically with the highly BuChE-selective inhibitor MF-8622 at concentrations varying between 15 and 170 μM.[44] Extracellular ACh levels were measured simultaneously without using a second ChEI by means of the sensitive microdialysis method of Cuadra et al.[45] At the highest MF-8622 concentration (170 μM), the ACh level increased 15-fold (from a 5 nM baseline value to 75 nM). This implies that ACh concentration in and around cholinergic synapses in the cortex might have increased from nanomolar to low micromolar levels. These values approach inhibitory concentrations for AChE,[46] which might affect glial BuChE activity.

Particularly interesting from the clinical point of view is the relative rate of inhibition shown by several ChEIs towards human erythrocytes (AChE) and plasma (BuChE), shown in Table 6.3. We can see that most inhibitors presently utilized for AD therapy are not selective for AChE; however, they all show various degrees of clinical efficacy. Considering the drastic decrease in AChE activity taking place in the brain of AD patients (reaching 5% AChE levels at autopsy in some regions) and the large pool of BuChE still available in both glia and neurons, it may not constitute an advantage for a ChEI to be selective for AChE. On the contrary, a good balance between AChE and BuChE inhibition should result in higher therapeutic efficacy.

Cholinesterase inhibition: a mechanism to slow down deterioration?

The beta-amyloid peptide (beta-A4), one of the major constituent proteins of neuritic plaques in the brain of AD patients, originates from a larger polypeptide called APP.[47] APP is widely distributed throughout the mammalian brain, including rat brain, with a prevalent neuronal localization.[48] APP can be processed by several alternative pathways. A secretory pathway is believed to generate non-amyloidogenic soluble derivatives (APPs) following cleavage within the beta-A4 segment.[49] Cholinergic agonists regulating processing and secretion of APPs by increasing, as demonstrated in vitro, protein kinase C (PKC) activity of target cells,[50,51] could potentially decrease the

levels of amyloidogenic derivatives. It has been suggested that long-term inhibition of ChE, leading to increased levels of synaptic ACh, may result in activation of normal APP processing in AD brain.[29] This effect could slow down the formation of amyloidogenic APP fragments. Lahiri et al,[52] using nerve cell cultures, found that the level of secretion of APP derivatives into conditioned media was inhibited by treatment with 100 µg/ml tacrine. Chong and Suh[53] found a dose-dependent effect of tacrine on APP processing. Tacrine at low concentrations (0.02–0.5 mM) enhanced, whereas concentrations above 0.5 mM blocked, APP 770 processing in vitro. Haroutunian et al[54] reported that 1 week of treatment with the ChEI phenserine modulated the levels of secreted beta-APP in the CSF of forebrain cholinergic lesioned rats, suggesting that secretion of beta-APP into the CSF and neurons can be influenced by ChEIs. To determine whether ChEIs could alter the release of APP in brain, superfused cortical slices of the rat were used,[55] following the method described by Nitsch et al.[50] Both short- and long-acting ChEIs were tested for their ability to enhance the release of non-amyloidogenic soluble derivatives of APP. These included physostigmine, heptastigmine and DDVP (dichlorvos, a metabolite of metrifonate) at concentrations producing ChE brain inhibitions ranging from 5% to 95%. All three ChEIs elevated the release of APPs to significantly above control levels.

With the use of two different doses of tacrine (0.5 μM and 0.1 μM), it has been found that only the lower dose elevates the release of APPs in the cortical slices, which supports the finding of Chong and Suh[53] of a dose-dependent modulation of APP secretion by AChE inhibition. A similar increase was observed after muscarinic receptor stimulation with bethanechol, supporting results from in vitro experiments.[51] The author's findings suggest that administration of ChEIs to AD patients, by increasing secretion of APP and inhibiting formation of specific APP mRNAs, may exert a neuroprotective effect, activating normal APP processing through a muscarinic mechanism by decreasing amyloid deposition in brain cells.[55]

The future of cholinesterase inhibitors in Alzheimer therapy

Cholinesterase inhibitors are the only drugs presently demonstrating efficacy in AD treatment. We are beginning to discern advantages as well as therapeutical limitations of these drugs. We should also consider new possibilities for wider clinical application and possible improvement of the cholinergic approach. As previously discussed, selectivity for AChE does not seem to be a prerequisite for clinical efficacy. On the contrary, it would be interesting to test a selective BuChE inhibitor in view of possible interactions with beta-A4 accumulation, plaque formation[37] and lack of side-effects. The implication of a proteolytic activity directly associated with AChE is still controversial. Recent evidence implies that a classic ChEI would not be effective with regard to APP metabolism unless associated in its molecule with a selective protease inhibitor function. A bifunctional compound could be designed to achieve this. Another interesting concept is the combination of two cholinergic functions in the same molecule, such as a ChEI with muscarinic (M1 or M3) agonist or antagonist (M2) properties or nicotinic agonist properties.[3]

Analysis of the outcome of present clinical trials poses new questions and outlines new research goals, challenging the limits of the present therapy with ChEIs:

1. To improve the effect size beyond the 5-point ADAS-Cog and 0.5 CIBIC level: is this a question of higher dose?

2. To improve drug delivery and dosage to avoid or delay 'wearing off' and tolerance effects in long-term treatment.

3. To understand why some ChEIs show symptomatic improvement while others seem to maintain patient conditions at baseline level (stabilizaton effect): differences in pharmacological effect between various drugs may be the key to developing new and more efficacious products.

4. To understand the relationship between cognitive and behavioural improvement, and ChE inhibition: are there major differences between drugs in this respect which could explain differences in clinical efficacy?

5. To test the effect of ChEIs on populations of aged individuals with minimal cognitive impairment at risk for developing AD: this approach might throw some light on the question of protective versus symptomatic effect of ChEIs.

References

1. Giacobini E. The cholinergic system in Alzheimer disease. Prog Brain Res 1990;84:321-32.

2. Giacobini E. Cholinesterase inhibitors: from preclinical studies to clinical efficacy in Alzheimer disease. In: Quinn D, Balasubramaniam AS, Doctor BP, Taylor P (eds). Enzymes of the Cholinesterase Family. New York: Plenum Press, 1995:463-9.

3. Giacobini E. Cholinesterase inhibitors do more than inhibit cholinesterase. In: Becker R, Giaconbini E eds. Alzheimer disease: from molecular biology to therapy. Boston: Birkhäuser, 1996:187-204.

4. Scali C, Giovannini MG, Bartolini L et al. Effect of metrifonate on extracellullar brain acetylcholine and object recognition in aged rats. Eur J Pharmacol 1997;325:173-80.

5. Davis KL,Mohs RS. Enhancement of memory processes in Alzheimer's disease with multiple-dose intravenous physostigmine. Am J Psychiatry 1982;139:1421-4.

6. Thal L, Fuld PA, Masur DM, Sharpless NS. Oral physostigmine and lecithin improve memory in Alzheimer disease. Ann Neurol 1983;13:491-6.

7. Summers WK, Majowski LV, Marsh GM, Tachiki K, Kling A. Oral tetrahydroaminoacridine in long-term treatment of senile dementia, Alzheimer type. N Engl J Med 1986;315:1241-5.

8. Summers WK, Viesselman JO, Marsh GM, Candelora K. Use of THA in treatment of Alzheimer-like dementia: pilot study in twelve patients. Biol Psychi 1981;26:145-53.

9. Shaw H, Bentley G. Some aspects of the pharmacology of morphine with special reference to its antagonism by 5-aminoacridine and other chemically related compounds. Med J Aust 1949;2:868-75.

10. Albin SM, Bunegin B, Massopust LC, Jannetta P. Ketamine-induced postanesthetic delirium attenuated by tetrahydroaminoacridine. Exp Neurol 1974;44:126-9.

11. Gordh T, Walin A. Potentiation of the neuromuscular effect of succinylcholine by tetrahydro-aminoacridine. Acta Anaesthiol Scand 1961;5:55-61.

12. Shaw H, Bentley G. Anticholinesterase properties of tetrahydroaminoacrine. Aust J Exp Biol 1953;31:573-8.

13. Heilbronn E. Inhibition of cholinesterase by tetrahydroaminoacrine. Acta Chem Scand 1961;15:1386-90.

14. Anand R, Hartman RD, Hayes PE. An overview of the development of SDZ ENA 713, a brain selective cholinesterase inhibitor. In: Becker R, Giacobini E, eds. Alzheimer disease: from molecular biology to therapy. Boston: Birkhäuser, 1996:239-43.

15. Farlow M, Gracon SI, Hershey LA, Lewis KW, Sadowski CH, Dolan-Ureno JA. Controlled trial of tacrine in Alzheimer's disease. JAMA 1992;268:2523-9.

16. Knapp MJ, Knopman DS, Solomon PR. A 30 week randomized controlled trial of high-dose tacrine in patients with Alzheimer's disease. JAMA 1994;271:985-91.

17. Roger SL, Friedhoff LT. The efficacy and safety of donepezil in patients with Alzheimer's disease: results of a US multicentre, randomized, double-blind, placebo-controlled trial. Dementia 1996;7:293-303.

18. Giacobini E, Becker R, McIlhany M, Kumar V. Interacerebroventricular administration of cholinergic drugs: preclinical trials and clinical experience in Alzheimer patients. In: Giacobini E, Becker R, eds. Current research in Alzheimer therapy. New York: Taylor and Francis, 1988:113-22.

19. Mattio T, McIlhany M, Giacobini E, Hallak M. The effects of physostigmine on acetylcholinesterase activity of CSF, plasma and brain. A comparison of intravenous and intraventricular administration in beagle dogs. Neuropharmacology 1986;25:1167-77.

20. Giacobini E, DeSarno P, Clark B, McIlhany M. The cholinergic receptor system of the human brain—neurochemical and pharmacological aspects in aging and Alzheimer. In: Nordberg A, Fuxe K, Holmstedt B, eds. Progress in brain research. Amsterdam: Elsevier, 1989:335-43.

21. Giacobini E, Cuadra G. Second and third generation cholinesterase inhibitors: From preclinical studies to clinical efficacy. In: Giacobini E, Becker R, eds. Alzheimer disease: therapeutic strategies. Boston: Birkhäuser, 1994:155-71.

22. Giacobini E. Cholinomimetic therapy of Alzheimer disease: does it slow down deterioration? In: Racagni G, Brunello N, Langer SZ, eds. Recent advances in the treatment of neurodegenerative disorders and cognitive dysfunction, vol. 7. Internatonal Academy of Biomedical Drug Research. New York: Karger, 1994:51-7.

23. Augustinsson KK. Cholinesterases. A study in comparative enzymology. Acta Physiol Scand 1948;15(suppl 52);1-182.

24. Giacobini E. From molecular structure to Alzheimer therapy. Jpn J Pharmacol 1997;74:225-41.

25. Becker E, Giacobini E. Mechanisms of cholinesterase inhibition in senile dementia of the Alzheimer type. Drug Dev Res 1988;12:163-95.

26. Becker R, Giacobini E. Pharmacokinetics and pharmacodynamics of acetylcholinesterase inhibition. Drug Dev Res 1988;14:235-46.

27. Gallo MA, Lawryk N. Organic phosphorus pesticides In: Hayes W, Laws E, eds. Handbook of pesticides toxicology. San Diego: Academic Press, 1991:927-9.

28. Bareggi SR, Giacobini E. Acetylcholinesterase activity in ventricular and cisternal CSF of dogs. J Neurosci Res 1978; 3:335-9.

29. Scarsella G, Toschi G, Bareggi SR, Giacobini E. Molecular forms of cholinesterase in cerebrospinal fluid, blood plasma and brain tissue of the beagle dog. J Neurosci Res 1979;4:19-24.

30. Elble R, Giacobini E, Scarsella GF. Cholinesterase in cerebrospinal fluid. Neurology 1987;44:403-7.

31. Rider JA, Moeller HC, Swader J, Weilerstein RW. The effect of parathion on human red blood cell and plasma cholinesterase. AMA Arch Ind Health Section II 1958;18:441-5.

32. Genina SA. Dynamics of blood cholinesterase activity in workers exposed to some organophosphorus insecticides during aerochemical

application. Gig Tr Prof Zabol 1974;12:42–4 (in Russian).

33. Silver A. The Biology of Cholinesterases. Agricultural Research Council Institute, New York: Elsevier, 1974:426–47.

34. Giacobini E, Holmstedt B. Cholinesterase content of certain regions of the spinal cord as judged by histochemical and cartesian diver technique. Acta Physiol Scand 1958;42:12–27.

35. Giacobini E. Distribution and localization of cholinesterases in nerve cells. Acta Physiol Scand 1959;45(suppl 156):1.

36. Giacobini E. Metabolic relations between glia and neurons studied in single cells. In: Maynard M, Cohen MD, Snider R, eds. Morphological and biochemical correlates of neural activity. New York: Harper & Row, 1964:15–38.

37. Wright CI, Geula C, Mesulam MM. Neuroglial cholinesterases in the normal brain and in Alzheimer's disease: relationship to plaques, tangles and patterns of selective vulnerability. Ann Neurol 1993;34:373–84.

38. Perry EK, Perry RH, Blessed G, Tomlinson BE. Changes in brain cholinesterases in senile dementia of Alzheimer type. Neuropathol Appl Neurobiol 1978;4:273–7.

39. Arendt T, Brückner MK, Lange M, Bigl V. Changes in acetylcholinesterase and butyrylcholinesterase in Alzheimer's disease resemble embryonic development—a study of molecular forms. J Neurochem Int 1992;21:381–96.

40. Davies P. Neurotransmitter-related enzymes in senile dementia of the Alzheimer type. Brain Res 1979;171:319–27.

41. Atack JR, Perry EK, Bonham JR, Candy JM, Perry RH. Molecular forms of butyrylcholinesterase in the human neocortex during development and degeneration of the cortical cholinergic system. J Neurochem 1987;48:1687–92.

42. Ogane N, Giacobini E, Messamore E. Preferential inhibition of acetylcholinesterase molecular forms in rat brain. Neurochem Res 1992;17:489–95.

43. Ogane N, Giacobini E, Struble R. Differential inhibition of acetylcholinesterase molecular forms in

normal and Alzheimer disease brain. Brain Res 1992;589:307–12.

44. Giacobini E, Griffini P.L, Maggi T, Mascellani G, Mandelli R. Butyrylcholinesterase: is it important for cortical acetylcholine regulation? Soc. Neurosci. 26th Annual Meeting, 1996, abstract 84.18.

45. Cuadra G, Summers K, Giacobini E. Cholinesterase inhibitor effects on neurotransmitters in rat cortes *in vivo*. J Pharmacol Exp Ther 1994;270:277–84.

46. Massoulié J, Toutant JP. Vertebrates ChEs: structure and types of interaction. In: Whittaker VP, ed. Handbook of Experimental Pharmacology, Vol 86, The cholinergic synapse. Berlin, Heidelberg: Springer Verlag, 1988:167–224.

47. Kang J, Lemaire H-G, Unterbeck A et al. The precursor of Alzheimer disease amyloid A4 protein resembles a cell-surface receptor. Nature 1987;325:733–6.

48. Beeson JG, Shelton ER, Chan HW, Gage FH. Differential distribution of amyloid protein precursor immunoreactivity in the rat brain studied by using five different antibodies. J Comp Neurol 1994;342:78–96.

49. Sisodia SS, Koo EH, Beyreuther K, Unterbeck A, Price DL. Evidence that beta amyloid protein in Alzheimer disease is not derived by normal processing. Science 1990;248:492–5.

50. Nitsch RM, Slack BE, Wurtman RJ, Growdon JH. Release of Alzheimer precursor derivatives stimulated by activation of muscarinic acetylcholine receptors. Science 1992;258:304–7.

51. Buxbaum JD, Oishi M, Chen Hl et al. Cholinergic agonists and interleukin 1 regulate processing and secretion of the Alzheimer βA4 amyloid protein precursor. Proc Natl Acad Sci USA 1992;89:10075–8.

52. Lahiri DK, Lewis S, Farlow MR. Tacrine alters the secretion of the beta-amyloid precursor protein in cell lines. J Neurosci Res 1994;37:777–87.

53. Chong YH, Suh YH. Amyloidogenic processing of Alzheimer's amyloid precursor protein in vitro and its modulation by metal ions and tacrine. Life Sci 1996;59:545–57.

54. Haroutunian V, Greig N, Pei XF et al. Pharmacological modulation of Alzheimer's b-amyloid precursor protein levels in the CSF of rats with forebrain cholinergic system lesions. Soc Neurosci 1996;22:1169.

55. Mori F, Lai CC, Fusi F, Giacobini E. Cholinesterase inhibitors increase secretion of APPs in rat brain cortex. Neurosci Rep 1995;6:633–6.

56. Canal I, Imbimbo BP. Clinical trials and therapeutics: relationship between pharmacodynamic activity and cognitive effects of eptastigmine in patients with Alzheimer's disease. Clin Pharmacol Ther 1996;15:49–59.

57. Imbimbo BP. Eptastigmine: a cholinergic approach to the treatment of Alzheimer's disease. In: Becker R, Giacobini E, eds. Alzheimer disease: from molecular biology to therapy. Boston: Birkhäuser, 1996:223–30.

58. Becker R, Markwell JA, Moriearty SJ, Unni LK, Vicari S. Double-blind, placebo-controlled study of metrifonate, an acetylcholinesterase inhibitor, for Alzheimer disease. Alzheimer Dis Assoc Disord 1996;10:124–31.

59. Becker R, Moriearty SJ, Unni L, Vicari S. Cholinesterase inhibitors as therapy in Alzheimer's disease: benefit to risk considerations in clinical

applications. In: Becker R, Giacobini E, eds. Alzheimer disease: from Molecular Biology to Therapy. Boston: Birkhauser, 1996:257–66.

60. Morris J, Cyrus P, Orazem J, Mas J, Bieber F, Gulanski B. Metrifonate: potential therapy for Alzheimer's disease. Am Soc Neurol Meeting, Boston, 1997 abstract 155.

61. Imbimbo BP, Lucchelli PE. A pharmacodynamic strategy to optimize the clinical response to eptastigmine. In: Becker R, Giacobini E, eds. Alzheimer disease: therapeutic strategies. Boston: Birkhauser, 1994:223–30.

62. Wilkinson D. Galanthamine hydrobromide— results of a group study. Eighth Congress Int Psychoger, Jerusalem 1997, Abstract p.70.

63. Becker R, Colliver J, Elbe R. Effects of metrifonate, a long-acting cholinesterase inhibitor. Drug Dev Res 1990;19:425–34.

64. Rogers SL, Doody R, Mohs R, Friedhoff LT. E2020 produces both clinical global and cognitive test improvement.Neurology 1996;46(abstract 217).

65. Rogers SL, Farlour M, Doody R et al. A 24-week, double-blind, placebo-controlled trial of donepezil in patients with Alzheimer's disease. Neurology 1998;50:136–45.

Classes of drugs

Albert Enz

7

Introduction

The heterogeneity of Alzheimer's disease (AD) and the presently incomplete state of pathophysiological knowledge are still serious challenges to the development of pharmacological therapies for this disease. However, many avenues have been opened recently by the progress which has been made in this direction. For example, the identification of neurochemical abnormalities in the brains of AD patients has led to pharmacotherapies. Until now these have been largely palliative and addressed at reducing symptoms. Nevertheless, it is reasonable to look forward in the future to the development of drugs that will be able to inhibit the evolution of the neuropathological alterations themselves which give rise to the symptoms. The palliative approach or type of therapy is mainly directed towards the neurotransmitter systems which are impaired in the disease and whose stimulation or rescue will result in improved cognitive functioning. Effective treatments for AD are a healthcare necessity for economic reasons and because of the severe toll this disease exacts on the quality of life of both patients and caregivers. Current research into new drugs is focused on agents that will prevent, slow down and/or halt the progress of the disease process.

Cholinergic drugs

The first major advance in understanding AD was the discovery that the network of cholinergic subcortical neurons projecting to the cerebral cortex and hippocampus was severely damaged in AD.[1,2] These projections represent key components playing an important role in attention and memory functions.[3] The extent of damage to these cholinergic projections correlates closely with the degree of the clinical state of AD and gave rise to the 'cholinergic hypotheses', according to which a large part of the memory impairment of AD is attributable to cholinergic hypofunction. Numerous attempts to develop a cholinergic replacement therapy have been developed based on this theory.

Acetylcholine precursors

Analogous to the activation of the dopaminergic system in Parkinson's disease, where the treatment is provided by the administration of the precursor L-DOPA, choline was administered in the form of choline or phosphatidylcholine (lecithin). The outcome was very little activation of the damaged system or even a worsening influence.[4,5]

Cholinergic agonists

The approach of stimulating directly the central cholinergic receptors by muscarinic agonists is based on the findings that the density of at least two subtypes, M1 and M2, is not changed in post-mortem brains of AD patients.[6] Initially, several drugs were tested clinically, such as arecoline,[7] pilocarpine,[8] bethanechol,[9] oxotremorine[10] and RS86,[11] but were discarded because of their peripheral or central cholinergic side-effects or short biological half-life. Since these early studies, more brain-selective muscarinic agonists with more receptor subtype selectivity have reached the stage of clinical investigation. For example, Xanomeline (LY 246708, Novo Nordisk/Lilly), a muscarinic agonist with a certain selectivity for the M1 receptor, has had some efficacy in phase II trials. The partial muscarinic agonist Milameline (CI-979, Parke-Davis/Roussel Uclaf) showed efficacy in phase II clinical trials but was found to lack efficacy in phase III trials. No data are currently available from clinical trials of another M1 selective agonist, YM 796 (Yamanouchi), or for the M1 selective compound SB 202026 from Smith Kline Beecham. The M1 agonist AF102B, also known as FK 508 (Snow Brand), has been under clinical investigation for a long time. This compound reportedly has an ideal profile from the preclinical point of view, including an influence on beta-amyloid production. However, in early clinical phases it has shown only small improvements in ADAS-Cog score.

Nicotinic agonists of interest for AD treatment are still in the preclinical stages, with the exception of Taiho's GTS 21, which is in phase I trials in Europe. Abbott's ABT-418, a nicotinic subtype selective agonist, has been discontinued.

Cholinesterase inhibitors

Acetylcholinesterase inhibitors (AChEIs) interact with the enzyme that metabolizes acetylcholine (ACh) in the synaptic cleft.[12] Their action is to maintain the availability of the transmitter ACh, which is reduced in AD brains. This class of anti-AD agents represents the only agents today which are approved for amelioration of the symptoms in this disease. A potential advantage of these agents, compared to muscarinic agonists, is that they better preserve spatiotemporal patterns of cholinergic activity, which may be important for learning and memory. The first report on improvement of cognitive function in AD patients by an AChEI, tetrahydroaminoacridine (tacrine), was published by Summers et al in 1986.[13] The compound was the first to be approved by the FDA, in 1996, and has been used therapeutically since 1997. The adverse effects of tacrine, mainly the elevation of the liver enzyme alanine aminotransferase, have limited the widespread use of this compound.[14] Donepezil (E2020, Eisai/Pfizer) is a selective reversible AChEI successfully introduced in 1997. The compound produces improvement in AD scales such as ADAS-Cog and CIBIC plus and has, at the clinical doses used (5 and 10 mg), only minor side-effects. Its long half-life (>70 h), partly due to its strong plasma protein binding, allows once-a-day dosing. SDZ ENA 713 (Rivastigmine, Novartis) inhibits cholinesterase pseudoirreversibly as a carbamate, establishing a long-lasting enzyme inhibition. In all pivotal clinical studies this compound gave significant improvements in different AD scales, including the scale for activities for daily living Progressive Deterioration Scale[15,16] (PDS). This drug has been in clinical use in Switzerland since 1997. Another potential drug can be seen in metrifonate (Bayer), which acts after its conversion into dichlorvos as an irreversible cholinesterase inhibitor. This compound is currently being investigated in phase III trials for its potential use in AD therapy. Many other AChEIs are also under development, such as the competitive inhibitor galanthamine (Shire, Jansen, Waldheim), which is presently in clinical phase III trials. A natural product, huperzine, also acts mainly as a cholinesterase inhibitor and has been used in traditional medicine for the geriatric population in China for a long time. Eptastigmine, a derivative of physostigmine without its disadvantages, has long-lasting effects and is under development in Italy by Mediolanum. This drug was co-developed by Mediolanum and Merck, Sharp and Dohme (MSD) until clinical phase II, but MSD withdrew following the occurrence of neutropenia in two patients.

In summary, this class of pharmacological agents seems for the time being to offer the most promising symptomatological treatment for AD.

Non-cholinergic drugs
Anti-inflammatory agents

The use of anti-inflammatory drugs in AD is based on evidence of activated inflammatory processes in AD brains which may contribute to the neurodegeneration, and on clinical and epidemiological observations concerning the effects of anti-inflammatory drugs. Co-localized with senile plaques and neurofibrillary tangles in AD brains are found immunoinflammatory molecules which could contribute to the pathological course of the disease.[17] Because neurons are non-dividing postmitotic cells, those which are killed by inflammatory attack cannot be replaced. There is evidence that treatment with nonsteroidal anti-inflammatory drugs can prevent or delay the onset of AD.[18-20] Generic drugs such as aspirin or indomethacin have, however, peripheral side-effects. Several clinical investigations support the idea that anti-inflammation therapy in AD may be beneficial.[21-24]

Antioxidants and radical scavengers

Based on the hypothesis that free radicals are involved in the damage of neurons following ischaemia or stroke and are among the weapons of activated inflammatory cells, drugs acting either as free radical scavengers or as antioxidants were proposed for therapeutic use in AD. The monoamine oxidase B (MAO-B) inhibitor/antioxidant selegiline had an influence on disease progression in moderately impaired AD patients, as did vitamin E (alpha-tocopherol). For both drugs the reported slowing of the progression of AD is attributed to their antioxidant properties.[25] Lazabemide (RO 19–6327, Roche) and other MAO-B inhibitors are currently undergoing clinical phase III evaluation for AD treatment. The selective MAO-A inhibitor moclobemide (Roche) has shown, in addition to its antidepressive action, a cognitive enhancing effect in geriatric patients[26] and has been proposed for further clinical investigations in AD.[27]

N-methly-D-aspartate (NMDA) antagonists

The potential use of antagonists of NMDA-type glutamate receptors is another hypothesis related to the inhibition of cytotoxic neurotransmitter systems. Excessive occurrence of excitatory amino acids in the synaptic cleft during neurotransmission can damage cells in the vicinity by acting through NMDA and alpha-amino-3-hydroxy-5-methyl-4-isoxazole-propionic acid (AMPA)/kainate receptors.[28] The interaction between AMPA/kainate and NMDA receptors is important in the lesion processes. Therefore, the clinical investigation of antagonists for these receptors has been advocated in the treatment of degenerative brain diseases. Several excitatory amino acid (EAA) antagonists (NMDA-type antagonists) are in development, and some of them are undergoing clinical trials such as remacemide (Astra), dizolcipine (MSD) and SDZ EAA 494 (Novartis).

Neurotrophic agents

Neurotrophins or trophic factors are peptides or peptidomimetics promoting the growth and survival of neurons. Nerve growth factor (NGF) enhances the survival of cholinergic basal forebrain cells in vitro and in vivo. In limited clinical studies in which NGF was added to the cerebrospinal fluid, modest improvement has been observed.[29] The search for smaller molecules mimicking neurotrophic activity is ongoing. Immunophilins, inhibitors of rotamase, are active in several animal models of neurodegeneration (GPI-1046, Guilford). Propentofylline (HWA-285, Hoechst

Marion-Roussel) is a phosphodiesterase inhibitor and an adenosine uptake inhibitor which is currently under investigation in AD patients (phase III trials).[30] This drug may interact with processes that induce brain cell death and therefore may contribute to slowing down the progression of the disease.[31]

Nootropics

The name 'nootropics' was applied to a class of compound structurally related to piracetam (UCB) and reported to facilitate learning and memory in some animal models. Included in this class are aniracetam (Roche),[32] pramiracetam and oxiracetam (Novartis).[33] The underlying mechanism of action of these drugs is unclear, but they may have effects on GABAergic neurotransmission, enhance the activation of AMPA-type glutamate receptors and also possibly possess EAA antagonistic properties. By interaction with a claimed central binding site, ACh can be released. These compounds are presently used in Europe and Japan only. Other drugs belonging to the class of nootropics are idebenone (Takeda) and indenoxanine (Yamanouchi). A further nootropic drug is the 'ampakine' CX-516 (Cortex Pharmaceuticals), acting as an enhancer of EAA neurotransmission by potentiating EAA action at AMPA-type

glutamate receptors. The drug is undergoing clinical phase II trials.

Drugs claimed to interact with APP processing

The majority of the previously described anti-AD drugs are used or envisaged for the treatment of symptoms of the disease. Currently, there is no cure or preventive treatment available for this disease. From ongoing basic research, however, hope arises that in the near future novel drugs will be discovered which either slow down the progression of the disease, prevent its onset or restore the functions already damaged. Current approaches are aimed at the reduction of the pathological hallmarks in the brain of AD, the amyloid-containing senile plaques and/or the tau-protein-associated senile tangles, or at reducing the neurotoxicity associated with these features. The neurotoxic amyloid-beta-peptide (Aβ) is a major component of the Alzheimer plaques. Its precursor protein (APP), a glycoprotein, is secreted from brain cells into the extra-cellular space and has important physiological roles. The formation of amyloid-containing senile plaques in AD brains is believed to be the result of abnormal processing of APP. The process by which Aβ is generated is known as endoproteolysis. Inhibition of the enzymes involved in Aβ formation, mainly proteases or cathepsin-like secretases, can prevent Aβ formation in vitro. Inhibitors known to date include certain TNF-α converting enzyme inhibitors, leupeptin, brefeldin A and bafilomycin. It is likely that such compounds have been identified and are in preclinical testing for their usefulness as therapeutic agents. Another approach is to search for compounds which form complexes with Aβ and thus prevent its aggregation into amyloid plaques. Compounds serving as candidates for such an action are, for example, Congo red and its analogue chrysamine G, anapsos, a plant product, and rifamicin, an antibiotic.

Outlook

The pharmacotherapy of AD based on the available drugs today is limited to the treatment of the symptoms of the disease, such as improvement and or maintenance of cognition, behaviour and activities of daily living. Although there are claims that some of these treatments may also influence the disease progression, no causal therapy is available. Ongoing research will hopefully supply in the near future drug treatments resulting in prevention and/or stabilization of this neurodegenerative disease, whose prevalence is still increasing.

References

1. Davies P. A critical review of the role of the cholinergic system in human cognition. Ann NY Acad Sci 1985;444:212-17.

2. Perry EK. The cholinergic hypothesis—ten years on. Br Med Bull 1986;42:63-9.

3. Collerton D. Cholinergic function and intellectual decline in Alzheimer's disease. Neuroscience 1986;19:1-28.

4. Giacobini E, Becker R. Present progress and future development in the therapy for Alzheimer's disease. Prog Clin Biol Res 1989;317:1121-54.

5. Davidson M, Stern RG, Bierer LM, et al. Cholinergic strategies in the treatment of Alzheimer's disease. Acta Psychiatr Scand Suppl 1991;366:47-51.

6. Palacios JM, Cortes R, Probst A, Karobath M. Mapping of subtypes of muscarinic receptors in the human brain with receptor autoradiographic techniques. Trends Pharmacol Sci 1986;6:56-60.

7. Tariot PN, Cohen RM, Sunderland T, Mellow AM. Multiple-dose arecoline infusion in Alzheimer's disease. Arch Gen Psychiatry 1988;45:901-4.

8. Caine ED. Cholinomimetic treatment fails to improve memory disorders. N Engl J Med 1980;315:1241-5.

9. Read S. Intracerebroventricular bethanechol: dose and response. In: Giacobini E, Becker R, eds. Current research in Alzheimer therapy. New York: Taylor and Francis, 1988:315-24.

10. Davis KL, Hollander E, Davidson M, Davis BM, Mohs RC, Horvath TB, Induction of depression with oxotremorine in patients with Alzheimer's disease. Am J Psychiatry 1987;144:469-71.

11. Hollander E, Davidson M, Mohs RC, et al. RS 86 in the treatment of Alzheimer's disease: cognitive and biological effects. Biol Psychiatry 1987;22:1067-78.

12. Giacobini E. Cholinomimetic therapy of Alzheimer's disease: does it slow down deterioration? In: Racagni G, Brunello N, Langer SZ, eds. Recent advances in the treatment of neurodegenerative disorders and cognitive dysfunction, Vol. 7. International Academy of Biomedical Drug Research, New York: Karger, 1994:51-7.

13. Summers K, Majovski LV, Marsh GM, Tachiki K, Kling A. Oral tetrahydroaminoacridine in long-term treatment of senile dementia, Alzheimer type. N Engl J Med 1986;315:1241-5.

14. Watkins PB, Zimmerman HJ, Knapp MJ, Gracon SI, Lewis KW. Hepatotoxic effects of tacrine administration in patients with Alzheimer's disease. JAMA 1994;271:992-8.

15. Anand R, Gharabawi G. Efficacy and safety results of the early phase studies with Exelon (ENA 713) in Alzheimer's disease: an overview. J Drug Dev Clin Pract 1996;8:109-16.

16. Brufani M, Filocamo L, Lappa S, Maggi A. New acetylcholinesterase inhibitors. Drugs Fut 1997;22:397-410.

17. Perlmutter LS, Barron E, Chui HC. Morphologic association between microglia and senile plaque amyloid in Alzheimer's disease. Neurosci Lett 1990;119:32-6.

18. Eikelenboom P, Zhan SS, van Gool WA, Allsop D. Inflammatory mechanisms in Alzheimer's disease. Trends Pharmacol Sci 1994;15:447-50.

19. McGeer PL, McGeer EG. In: Khachaturian ZS, Radebough TS, eds. Alzheimer's disease. Cause(s), diagnosis, treatment and care. Boca Raton FL: CRC Press, 1996:217-25.

20. Rogers J, Conceptual issues in research on inflammation and Alzheimer's disease. In: Brioni J, Decker MW, eds. Pharmacological treatment of Alzheimer's disease: Molecular and neurobiological foundations. New York: Wiley-Liss, 1997:493-502.

21. Rich JB, Rasmusson DX, Folstein MF, Carson KA, Kawas C, Brandt J. Nonsteroidal anti-inflammatory drugs in Alzheimer's disease. Neurology 1995;45:51-5.

22. Beard CM, Kokman E, Kurland LT. Rheumatoid arthritis and susceptibility to Alzheimer's disease. Lancet 1991;337:1426.

23. Breitner JC, Gau BA, Welsh KA, et al. Inverse association of anti-inflammatory treatments and Alzheimer's disease: initial results of a co-twin control study. Neurology 1994;44:227-32.

24. Rogers J, Kirby LC Hempelman SR, et al. Clinical trial of indomethacin in Alzheimer's disease. Neurology 1993;43:1609-11.

25. Sano M, Ernesto C, Thomas RG, et al. A controlled trial of selegiline, alpha tocopherol, or both as treatment for Alzheimer's disease. N Engl J Med 1997;336:1216-22.

26. Pancheri P, Delle-Chiaie R, Donnini M, et al. Effects of moclobemide on depressive symptoms and cognitive performance in a geriatric population: a controlled comparative study versus imipramine. Clin Neuropharmacol 1994;17(suppl 1):S58-73.

27. Chan-Palay V. Depression and senile dementia of the Alzheimer type: a role for moclobemide. Psychopharmacology 1992;106:S137-9.

28. Farouqui AA, Horrocks LA. Excitatory amino acid receptors, neural membrane phospholipid metabolism and neurological disorders. Brain Res Rev 1991;16:171-91.

29. Seiger A, Nordberg A, von Holst H, et al. Intracranial infusion of purified nerve growth factor to an Alzheimer patient: a first attempt of a possible future treatment strategy. Behav Brain Res 1993;57:255-61.

30. Kittner B, Rössner M, Rother M. Clinical trials in dementia with propentofyeline. Ann NY Acad Sci 1997;826:337-347.

31. Schubert P, Ogata T, Rudolphi K et al. Support of homeostatic glial cell signaling: a novel therapeutic approach by propentofyeline. Ann NY Acad Sci 1997;826:337-347.

32. Lee CR, Benfield P. Aniracetam: an overview of its pharmacodynamic and pharmacokinetic properties, and a review of its therapeutic potential in senile cognitive disorders. Drugs Aging 1994;4:257-73.

33. Bottini G, Vallar G, Cappa S, et al. Oxiracetam in dementia: a double-blind, placebo-controlled study. Acta Neurol Scand 1992;86:237-41.

Pharmacoeconomic evaluation of new treatments for Alzheimer's disease

Bernie J O'Brien

8

Introduction

In recent years there has been marked growth in the application of economic evaluation methods to healthcare interventions in general, and to pharmaceuticals in particular.[1] In addition to the demonstration that a new medication is both safe and effective, jurisdictions such as Australia[2] and Ontario, Canada[3] now require economic evaluation defining 'value for money' before granting reimbursement status to new pharmaceuticals prescribed under publicly funded programs. Similar concerns have been voiced in the USA both in terms of reimbursement for interventions under federal programs such as Medicare[4] and, more recently, in the context of managed care. The two aims of this chapter are: (1) to introduce the basic principles of economic evaluation as they apply to pharmaceuticals, so-called 'pharmacoeconomics', and (2) to examine some of the issues that arise in conducting pharmacoeconomic evaluations of new drug treatments for Alzheimer's disease.

What is pharmacoeconomics?

Pharmacoeconomics is a relatively new term for a set of evaluative methods that have existed for many years. In essence, it is the application of economic evaluation methods such as cost-effectiveness and cost–benefit analysis to pharmaceuticals. There is a growing body of literature on methods for economic evaluation in health care, including textbooks,[5] guides in the medical literature[6,7] and government guidelines in both the USA[8] and Canada.[9]

The rationale for economic evaluation is twofold. First, the market for health care is unlike that for other commodities and services, where supply and demand are brought together through a price mechanism. In the absence of a functioning market, governments intervene (to differing degrees in different countries) to deliver or finance health care. Second, faced with a scarce and finite pool of resources, and in the absence of market price signals of what consumers' value, how should a government or the collective decision-making body (e.g. a formulary committee) allocate healthcare resources between the many competing demands? Fundamental to the economist's perspective on this dilemma of

choice is an understanding of the notion of *opportunity cost*, where the costs of implementing program A are the health benefits of an alternative program (B) that can no longer be pursued. The economist's definition of efficiency is an extension of this notion of opportunity cost. Using a simple production analogy of resource inputs and health benefit inputs, the pursuit of efficiency is an attempt to identify and reallocate resources to those healthcare interventions that offer the greatest health returns from our scarce resources. It is with this goal in mind that various techniques for economic evaluation have been developed.

Distinguishing features of economic evaluations

A full economic evaluation is comparative and considers both costs and effectiveness of alternatives. Therefore, economic appraisal is only as good as the epidemiologic and clinical data upon which it is based—it requires the comparison of outcomes and costs with some alternative (control group), as is common in any high-quality clinical study such as prospective randomized trials. Furthermore, economic evaluations should not be confused with cost-cutting or cost-containment. It is not about finding the 'cheapest' therapy independent of outcomes. A study that considers only costs offers little information which is relevant for defining value and improving the efficiency of resource allocation. A new therapy can still be deemed 'cost-effective' if it increases costs but improves patient outcomes, the focus being on the cost of additional units of benefits.[10]

The four main types of economic appraisal are listed in Table 8.1. For all methods of economic evaluation, direct costs refer to the value of resources consumed in delivering care (e.g. medicines, hospital days). The question of which costs to include will depend upon the viewpoint of the analysis (e.g. hospital, payer, society). From a societal viewpoint we may also wish to include productivity costs, these being the value of lost (or gained) production due to a patient's or caregiver's (in)ability to work or engage in other normal activities as a consequence of disease or treatment. The factors that differentiate the various methods of evaluation are the ways in which outcomes are quantified and valued.

Cost-minimization analysis (CMA)

If there is evidence that health outcomes from any intervention are equivalent to, or better than, the comparison therapy, it is legitimate to compare only costs. For example, Shapiro et al[11] demonstrated the cost savings associated with antibiotic prophylaxis with a more expensive drug regimen in abdominal and vaginal hysterectomy by virtue of the reduced risk and cost of managing subsequent postoperative infection. If a new intervention were demonstrated to be both less costly and more effective, it would have economic dominance (a 'win–win' situation), and should be adopted. An example of such economic dominance is the treatment to eradicate the bacterium *Helicobacter pylori* in the management of peptic ulcer disease: patients have fewer recurrences of ulcer and the overall cost is lower.[12]

Cost-effectiveness analysis (CEA)

For most new medicines the circumstance arises where the new treatment is both more costly and more effective than current therapy. CEA proceeds by identification of a single outcome of interest (e.g. reduced mortality) and expresses the incremental cost (treatment minus control) of achieving the incremental benefit. For example, in a study examining cholestyramine for lowering blood

Table 8.1
Features of the different forms of economic evaluation.

Type of economic evaluation	Measurement/ valuation of costs in both alternatives	Consequences	Measurement/ valuation of consequences
Cost-minimization	Money	Identical in all relevant respects	None
Cost-effectiveness	Money	Single effect, common to alternatives, but achieved to different degrees	Natural units (e.g. years of life gained, units of blood pressure reduction)
Cost–utility	Money	Single or multiple effects not necessarily common to the two alternatives; common effects may be achieved to different degrees	'Healthy days' or (more often) 'quality-adjusted life-years'
Cost–benefit	Money	Single or multiple effects, not necessarily common to the two alternatives; common effects may be achieved to different degrees	Money (e.g. consumers' willingness-to-pay)

cholesterol in middle-aged males, Oster and Epstein[13] estimated the cost per year of life gained to be $76 500.

A limitation of CEA is that health outcomes are often multidimensional, encompassing changes in both survival and health-related quality of life (HRQL): in this circumstance, either cost–utility analysis (CUA) or cost–benefit analysis (CBA) may be the preferred analytic tool.

Cost–utility analysis (CUA)

CUA differs from CEA because some attempt is made to resolve trade-offs between multiple outcomes such as mortality and HRQL. To conduct a CUA, data are required on health-related quality of life and preferences of health-care consumers for different combinations of health outcomes. One approach to this problem has been to construct a single index of composite outcomes known as quality-adjusted life-years (QALYs).[14] The logic of the QALY is to quantify preference or utility weights for health outcomes on a scale from death (= 0) to perfect health (= 1), and these are then used to adjust time periods of reduced health status in the summation of survival experience. For example, 10 years in a state of health judged to be 50% of normal quality would become 5 QALYs (10 × 0.5). There are several ways in which the quality weights can be estimated.[14]

Cost–benefit analysis (CBA)

Although this is the oldest and most widely practised method of economic evaluation in other sectors of public spending such as environment and transport, its application in health care has been problematic, largely because of the difficulties in attaching monetary values to health program outcomes.[15]

Application of CBA in strict accordance with its theoretical foundation in principles of welfare economics requires a determination of consumers' money valuations for expected health improvements using either observed or stated willingness-to-pay.[16] While such studies are technically feasible and have been undertaken in health care,[17-19] many researchers and policy-makers still view the application of CBA in the healthcare environment as experimental and requiring further development, particularly on issues of measurement.[20]

Pharmacoeconomics and Alzheimer's disease

Although some analysts have estimated the economic burden of AD[21,22] there have been very few pharmacoeconomic studies to date that evaluate the cost-effectiveness of new treatments for AD: this simply reflects the absence of new effective pharmaceutical therapies. The one exception is tacrine (Cognex), where two modeling studies from the USA have suggested that use of this drug will reduce overall costs by reducing and/or delaying admission to nursing homes or other long-term-care facilities.[23,24] The limited number of pharmacoeconomic studies and claims is set to change as many new compounds are marketed in the next few years. Already, donepezil (Aricept) has been launched in the USA and Canada, with a daily price tag of $4.59 in Canada. A central proposition of all economic analyses of these products is likely to be that slowing the rate of cognitive decline results in 'downstream' cost savings from delayed nursing home admissions which completely or partly offset the increased cost of daily drug therapy. What cost and effectiveness evidence do we need from such studies to address this and allied hypotheses? In the remainder of this chapter, some choices on these issues will be reviewed from the perspective of an analyst constructing a pharmacoeconomic evaluation in AD.

Choice 1: Which comparator?

For informed policy, we need evidence on the costs and effects of the new therapy compared to the most widely used existing therapy for the target patient population. Of course, what constitutes standard or usual care may vary by jurisdiction. For example, tacrine is not approved for use in Canada but is approved in the USA. Furthermore, healthcare payers will be acutely aware that a new drug may not ultimately be used as a substitute for an existing drug but as a complementary therapy. For this latter circumstance, a relevant economic study would probe the adjunctive effect and cost of the new drug in combination with others. A difficulty is that clinical trials designed for drug licensing will probably be placebo-controlled and will not deliver head-to-head evidence of comparative efficacy. (For a discussion of this general problem, see O'Brien.[25])

Choice 2: Which patient population?

Prior to the market launch of a new drug, the only available data are from controlled clinical trials. Typically, persons with particular comorbidities are excluded from such trials so that the drug can be studied in a well-defined population. Unfortunately, when the drug is used in real-world clinical practice, the treated population will not replicate the trial population and will present with comorbid conditions, often leading to a 'dilution' of the treatment effect seen in the trial. This contributes to the difference between the efficacy and effectiveness of a treatment. Economic evaluation is concerned with effectiveness (i.e. real-world use and outcomes) and may not be well served by trial-based efficacy data. Of course, the reality is that, at the time of marketing, phase III trial data are the best available. The issue is that the economic performance of a drug should be revisited in post-marketing studies to validate the pre-marketing predictions.

Choice 3: What viewpoint?

As noted above, the viewpoint adopted in a study dictates which costs and effects to include in the analysis. A very restricted viewpoint would be a simple balance sheet of drug costs— the viewpoint of the formulary or pharmacy manager. But such a viewpoint is patently ludicrous for most diseases and particularly AD. At minimum, for most settings such as managed care in the USA or a provincial Ministry of Health in Canada, we would want to take the perspective of the healthcare payer to capture any 'downstream' cost savings associated with reduced need for nursing home care. But even this viewpoint may systematically underestimate the resource consequences of AD and its treatment, which extend beyond the formal healthcare sector. Hence, a societal viewpoint would be comprehensive and seek to estimate costs of caregiving time and loss of work— whether paid or unpaid—and other resource use that may be paid for from other public purses such as social services.

Choice 4: What outcomes over what time horizon?

Given that AD is a chronic progressive disease with numerous symptoms arising largely out of decline in cognitive function, the measure of outcome for an economic evaluation of a treatment should be comprehensive in capturing the long-term health effects of treatment. However, the typical AD product licensing trial has an array of scales aimed at measuring cognitive function, typically over a relatively short duration (e.g. 24 weeks). This information is restrictive for the economic analysis in two ways. First, in the context of a treatment study, one would like to quantify the relation between cognitive function and factors such as activities of daily living (ADL) and broaden the concept of health or dysfunction under study. By extension, although formal measurement of HRQL may be infeasible in many AD subjects, such measurement may be desirable and informative among caregivers. Hence, the health impact of treatment and its measurement may legitimately extend beyond the AD patient. Indeed, a predictable irony that arises from this consideration is that alleviation of caregiver burden by admission of the AD patient to a nursing home (typically seen as a 'bad outcome') may actually improve quality of life for a caregiver.

The second issue is how to project long-term decline in cognitive function beyond the short-term treatment effect data from a trial. Such projection is desirable for economic analysis in AD, where a key issue is the extent to which treatment effectively delays admission to costly care environments such as nursing homes. In the absence of the ideal—long-term randomized studies that observe patients until nursing home admissions—there are two modeling strategies available. The first strategy would be to identify an existing longitudinal (i.e. cohort) study of AD subjects and conduct secondary analysis to determine the 'trajectory' of cognitive decline as a function of subjects' clinical and demographic characteristics. The treatment effect data from the trial can then be applied to such cohort data to extrapolate treatment and cohort group cognitive function. This approach has been used in a US economic model of donepezil[26] using the CERAD cohort study of AD.[27] A second approach is to use a statistical modeling technique known as Markov modeling,[28,29] which uses the observed cognitive change (over baseline) in the placebo group of the treatment trial as a means of predicting cognitive function (for treatment and control group) in the next period of time. We have recently used this approach in a Canadian economic model of donepezil.[30] Both approaches have strengths and weaknesses.

Choice 5: How to identify, measure and value costs?

The identification of relevant costs for an evaluation has already been discussed under viewpoint (choice 3) and time horizon (choice 4). But the measurement of resources used and how these should be valued raises problems. First, for reliable measurement, through time, of healthcare and other costs associated with different levels of cognitive functioning, one will need to look beyond the short-term product registration trial. Data on resource use may be available from longitudinal or cross-sectional studies. An example of cross-sectional data is the study by Ernst et al,[31] who collected cost data in a small ($n = 64$) survey of AD patients and caregivers in California. Using regression modeling techniques, they estimated the relationship between a measure of cognitive function, the Mini-Mental State Examination (MMSE) score, and cost. Using this information they produced a predictive model relating change in MMSE (via some hypothetical treatment) to costs or savings in the future (Table 8.2). By similar reasoning, in the Canadian economic evaluation of donepezil,[30] data from the Canadian Study on Health and Aging (CSHA)[32] were used to estimate costs for MMSE ranges for persons with AD. The advantages of CSHA data is that they are representative of the population, the sample size is larger, and they also include details on caregiver time.

Once resource consumption has been measured for AD subjects with differing levels of cognitive function, it is necessary to attach dollar values to these resources. Although this is relatively straightforward for many healthcare resources, it is problematic for informal care, where no actual expenditure may be incurred. One option is to estimate the market value of replacing the caregiver's contributions with hired help—the so-called 'replacement cost' method. Another approach is to value the time of the caregiver as being equal to what they would earn in the labor market—the 'opportunity cost' method (see Drummond et al[6] for details). The value of caregiver's time is likely to be a central methodologic issue for AD treatment studies in the future. Allied to this is the ongoing methodologic debate concerning the valuation of time lost from work. For example, in the presence of an excess supply of labor (i.e. unemployment), if a worker is 'lost' because they must stay home as a caregiver, that person's production is lost not until retirement age, but up until the point where they can be replaced by another person (the so-called friction cost method).[33]

Concluding remarks

This chapter is an introduction to the basic principles of economic evaluation as they are applied to pharmaceuticals (pharmacoeconomic), and a review of some of the problems and issues that arise when designing such evaluative studies for new AD drugs. In the absence of long-term, post-marketing, head-to-head comparison, by randomized economic trials with a range of relevant health outcomes for patients and caregivers, we must do the best we can with available data. Given that the rationale of many economic studies

Table 8.2
Estimated annual savings (US dollars) in direct and total costs per patient with Alzheimer's disease by changes in MMSE scores.[22,31]

Initial MMSE Score	Savings if MMSE score is raised by average annual point totals ($)				Savings if MMSE score is prevented from falling by average annual point totals ($)			
	+10	+5	+2	+1	-1	-2	-5	-10
20	1 965	1242	587	312	356	765	2424	7 537
15	3 666	2424	1186	638	744	1611	5113	13 733
12	5 630	3805	1876	1008	1164	2494	7407	16 125
7	11 213	7407	3418	1770	1846	3706	8718	–
5	13 733	8619	3706	1860	1806	3494	7429	–
2.04	16 111	8733	3219	1526	1324	2434	–	–

will be to predict long-term cost savings from reduced nursing home admissions in the future, a major area of research will be in using longitudinal AD data and statistical models to extrapolate from short-term trials to long-term effectiveness and costs. A second major area of methodologic controversy, which is central to AD treatment evaluation, is how caregiver time and quality of life should be factored into the public policy debate on value for money from AD treatment.

Acknowledgment

Dr O'Brien is the recipient of a career award in Health Sciences from the Prescription Drug Manufacturer's Association and Medical Research Council of Canada.

References

1. Elixhauser A, Luce BR, Taylor WR, et al. Health care CBA/CEA: an update in the growth and composition of the literature. Med Care 1993;31:js1-11.

2. Commonwealth of Australia: Guidelines for the pharmaceutical industry on preparation of submissions to the Pharmaceutical Benefits Advisory Committee: including submissions involving economic analyses (Department of Health, Housing and Community Services, 1990).

3. Detsky AS. Guidelines for preparation of economic analysis of pharmaceutical products: a draft document for Ontario and Canada. Pharmacoeconomics 1993;3:354-61.

4. Leaf A. Cost-effectiveness as a criterion for Medicare coverage. N Engl J Med 1989;321:898-900.

5. Drummond MF, O'Brien BJ, Stoddart GL, Torrance GW. Methods for the economic evaluation of health care programmes. Oxford: Oxford University Press, 1997.

6. Drummond MF, Richardson WS, O'Brien BJ, et al, for the Evidence-based Medicine Working Group: Users' Guides to the Medical Literature XIII. How to use an article on economic analysis of clinical practice. Part A. Are the results of the study valid? JAMA 1997;277:1552-7.

7. O'Brien BJ, Heyland D, Richardson WS, Levine M, Drummond MF: Users' Guides to the Medical Literature XIII. How to use an article on economic analysis of clinical practice: Part B: what are the results and will they help me in caring for my patients? JAMA 1997;277:1802-6.

8. Russell LB, Gold MR, Seigel JE, Daniels N, Weinstein MC. The role of cost-effectiveness analysis in health and medicine. JAMA 1996;276:1172-7.

9. Canadian Coordinating Office for Health Technology Assessment. Guidelines for economic evaluation of pharmaceuticals: Canada. 1st edn. Ottawa: CCOHTA, 1994.

10. Doubilet P, Weinstein MC, McNeil BJ. Use and misuse of the term 'cost-effective' in medicine. N Engl J Med 1986;314:253-355.

11. Shapiro M, Schoenbaum SC, Tager IB, Munoz A, Polk BF. Benefit–cost analysis of anti-microbial prophylaxis in abdominal and vaginal hysterectomy. JAMA 1983;249:1290-4.

12. O'Brien BJ, Goeree RA, Mohamed H, Hunt R. Cost-effectiveness of *Helicobacter pylori* eradication for the long-term management of duodenal ulcer in Canada. Arch Intern Med 1995;155:1958-64.

13. Oster G, Epstein AM. Cost-effectiveness of anti-hyperlipemic therapy in the prevention of coronary

heart disease. The case of cholestyramine. JAMA 1987;258:2381-7.

14. Torrance GW, Feeny D. Utilities and quality-adjusted life years. Int J Tech Assess Health Care 1989;5:559-75.

15. Johannesson M, Jonsson B. Economic evaluation in health care: is there a role for cost-benefit analysis? Health Policy 1991;17:1-23.

16. Gafni A. Using willingness-to-pay as a measure of benefits: what is the relevant question to ask in the context of public decision making? Med Care 1991;29:1246-52.

17. Thompson MS. Willingness-to-pay and accept risks to cure chronic disease. Am J Public Health 1986;76:392-6.

18. Johannesson M, Jonnsson B. Willingness to pay for antihypertensive therapy—results of a Swedish pilot study. J Health Econ 1991;10:461-74.

19. Appel LJ, Steinberg EP, Powe NR, Anderson GF, Dwyer SA, Faden RR. Risk reduction from low osmolality contrast media. What do patients think it is worth? Med Care 1990;28:324-34.

20. O'Brien BJ, Viramontes JL. Willingness-to-pay: a valid and reliable measure of health state preference. Med Decision Making 1994;14:289-97.

21. Østbye T, Crosse E. Net economic costs of dementia in Canada. Can Med Assoc J 1994;151:1457-64.

22. Ernst RL, Hay AJ. The US economic and social costs of Alzheimer's disease revisited. Am J Public Health 1994;84:1261-4.

23. Henke CJ, Birchmore MJ. The economic impact of tacrine in the treatment of Alzheimer's disease. Clin Ther 1997;19:330-44.

24. Lubeck DP, Mazonson PD, Bowe T. Potential effect of tacrine on expenditures for Alzheimer's disease. Med Interface 1997;October: 130-8.

25. O'Brien B. Economic evaluation of pharmaceuticals: Frankenstein's monster or vampire of trials? Med Care 1996;34:DS99-108.

26. Neumann PJ, Kuntz KM, Hermann RC, et al. The cost-effectiveness of donepezil in the treatment of mild or moderate Alzheimer's disease. Med Decision Making 1997;17:532(abstract).

27. Morris JC, Heyman A, Mohs RC, et al. The consortium to establish a registry for Alzheimer's disease. Neurology 1989;39:1159-65.

28. Sonnenberg F, Beck JR. Markov models in medical decision making: a practical guide. Med Decision Making 1993;13:322-38.

29. Beck JR, Pauker SG. The Markov process in medical prognosis. Med Decision Making 1983;3:419-58.

30. O'Brien BJ, Goeree RA, Hux M, et al. Economic evaluation of donepezil for the treatment of mild-to-moderate Alzheimer's disease in Canada. Alzheimer Dis Assoc Disord (submitted).

31. Ernst RL, Hay JW, Fenn C, Tinklenberg J, Yesavage JA. Cognitive function and the cost of Alzheimer disease. Arch Neurol 1997;54: 687-93.

32. Canadian Study of Health and Aging Working Group. The Canadian Study of Health and Aging: Risk factors for Alzheimer's disease in Canada. Neurology 1994;44:2073-80.

33. Koopmanschap MA, Rutten FFH, van Ineveld BM, van Roijen L. The friction cost method for measuring indirect costs of disease. J Health Econ 1995;14:171-89.

Social and ethical considerations

Stephen G. Post

9

The clinical ethics of the introduction of new anti-dementia compounds for Alzheimer disease's (AD) must be approached cautiously, because there are few outcome data available. Nevertheless, some social and ethical concerns are identifiable.

Five concerns are raised here. First, are placebo-control studies in anti-dementia drug development no longer morally acceptable? Second, is the introduction of an anti-dementia drug necessarily going to enhance quality of life for the individual and caregivers who have already navigated certain difficult adjustments? Third, at what point, if any, in the progression of AD would the application of an anti-dementia compound be considered unacceptable? Fourth, is there the possibility of the protraction of morbidity? Fifth, how will quality of life for caregiver and patient be balanced with the emerging analyses suggesting that compounds may save public costs by delaying nursing home placement?

The use of placebo controls

Codes of human subject research ethics indicate that once a treatment is reasonably established as an effective standard of care, experimental treatments must be evaluated in comparison with said standard. Under such circumstances, the control arm of a study must involve patients who are being treated with the proven efficacious compound. From an ethical perspective, this comparison of compounds insures that no patients will be denied benefits by virtue of relegation to a placebo-control population.

For researchers, while the design and analysis of comparative studies are more complex than those of placebo studies, this complexity is required by the principle of beneficence. For pharmaceutical companies, a further inconvenience is that new compound A may be proven effective, but perhaps not as much so as the competitor's compound B, against which A was compared. But nevertheless, the ethical superiority of non-placebo comparative studies must be asserted and implemented in order to remain consistent with a commitment to the good of patients.

At this point in time, no anti-dementia compound has been demonstrated to be sufficiently effective so as to make placebo-control studies in this field unethical. The outcome studies on anti-dementia compounds have, in fact, given rise to controversy. In some countries, a compound might be approved, while in others it is not; in some regions of a country, a given approved compound may or may not be used; geriatricians may find no clinical benefit in using a compound, while neurologists may find it of greater interest. Debates about interpretation of statistical improvements on mini-mental examinations are rampant, and critics of the new drugs are quick to distinguish statistical variations of several points on such examinations from a global clinical assessment of a patient's wellbeing.

Given the increased number of patients who must be recruited into non-placebo clinical trials, the questionable efficacy of existing compounds, and the complexities of assessing efficacy outside of a placebo control, the imposition of comparative studies at this time would be premature.

Living through the same adjustment twice

The introduction of any compound that relieves the symptoms of AD is immensely important and hopeful, given the dreadful effects of dementia on individuals, families, and society. However, in the cases of people with AD who have already become more than mildly demented, decisions to apply new compounds must be made individually and may need to be quickly reversed based on an assessment of quality of life. Most AD caregivers will not hesitate before trying new compounds. As one caregiver proclaimed during an Alzheimer's Association chapter meeting in Cleveland, 'I'm knee deep in my wife's diapers and I'll try anything!' But once the compound is applied, its impact must be carefully considered, with the possibility of its withdrawal.

On the positive side, a person with AD may for a period recover some degree of self-identity, or feel a brief liberation from the isolation of speech limitations. For example, a patient can say— and her family concurs—that she can now, with the help of a new compound, find more words. In another case, a woman who was too forgetful to cook any more regained sufficient memory to begin cooking again in relative safety (although one worries). The benefits of new

compounds will become clearer with clinical experience, although it is surely inappropriate to speak yet of any 'awakening' from AD.[1]

On the negative side, in patients already significantly demented, the application of an anti-dementia compound may be a mixed blessing with respect to quality of lives for both patient and caregiver. It is worth recalling the mixed impact of L-DOPA in some Parkinson patients. One of Oliver Sacks' patients, Miss D., after refusing the drug based on her self-assessment of quality of life, asserts: 'That L-DOPA, that stuff should be given its proper name— Hell-DOPA.'[2]

Temporary partial 'awakenings' with anti-dementia compounds in the context of an irreversible progressive dementing condition such as AD raise enormous ethical issues. In such cases, the patient and caregivers who have already navigated certain crises of cognitive decline may have to do so all over again. For example, the individual who has lost insight into his or her loss of capacity may be awakened into renewed insight and therefore into renewed anxiety; or the individual who has experienced aggressive behavioral problems that have since been successfully treated may, under the influence of an anti-dementia compound, revisit these problems. For AD patients who have already adjusted to significant decline, the sudden intrusion of a temporary awakening may or may not enhance quality of life; for caregivers, some of the most taxing phases of care may have to be virtually repeated.

None of the above-mentioned concerns with repetition of difficult adjustments pertain to the patient who is placed on an anti-dementia compound from very early on in the disease, hopefully on initial diagnosis. In such cases, patients will in many cases retain insights and capacities longer through the mild and moderate phases of AD. Thus, quality of life is extended by symptom mitigation despite the absence of any affect on the underlying process of neurologic deterioration. While the losses of significant thresholds of capacity will come, they will come more slowly, and the patient will need to adjust to them only once.

In this section, the questions are directed exclusively at those patients who have adjusted to their condition and, with the application of an anti-dementia compound, must eventually readjust. To clarify this concern, three recently collected cases will be presented. The first case account came over the author's e-mail system (23 June 1997) through the Cleveland Area Chapter of the Alzheimer's Association.

Case 1: 'Family story'

'At last night's Shaker Heights–Mt Pleasant support group, the subject of an anti-dementia drug came up. One caregiver (Dorothy A., daughter) brought the doctors prescription for the drug to the meeting and said she wasn't sure if she wanted to give it to her mom. Through the beautiful group process, they helped her decide what to do! You could see the relief on her face, and the decision ended up being no. Fortunately she had already discussed the pro's and con's of the drug with her brother, and was ready to come to a decision once more input had been received. But one family's story was especially moving, and is one that you might want to include in your study . . . Katie S. (wife) shared with Dorothy how much the drug has changed the situation with her husband. He is once again obsessing about finances, whereas before the drug, he had finally gotten to the point where he wasn't aware anymore—which was a relief for the family. He was very frustrated and suspicious about the financial situation earlier in the disease. Also, Katie shared that the children can no longer come over and talk openly about their problems and issues at home and with their own families, because he is now aware enough to be concerned and start worrying again. You might want to follow up with her and get the whole story, and hear the good aspects too.

Let me know how/if I can be of assistance. C.K.'

Case 1: Comment

The above case indicates how complex the decisions to place an already seriously demented patient on an anti-dementia compound can be. Symptoms are temporarily mitigated and a degree of insight is regained. On the other hand, intense anxiety is also regained. Are these limited but significant awakenings beneficent? As the author has argued in a recent book, if there is one kind point in the progression of AD, it may be when the patient comes to the point of forgetting that he or she forgets, because it is precisely at this point that the anxiety of insight into self-loss subsides.[3]

Case 2: 'A mute man speaks'

This second case emerged from discussion with the wife, Mrs K., of an elderly man who is quite advanced in his AD, to the point of not having spoken a word for a year. Mr K. has already been through the stage of behavioral problems, during which he exhibited considerable aggression and agitation. After behavioral medications and strenuous caregiving, he is now past this stage. He is described as mute, largely sedentary, and expressionless, although still able to eat with some assistance. He lives at home and his wife remains convinced that there is more of her husband left than the observer might think.

In this advanced condition of dementia, Mr K. was given a new drug at the recommendation of his neurologist. It never occurred to the neurologist or to Mrs K. that prescribing an anti-dementia compound might not enhance Mr K.'s or Mrs K.'s wellbeing. Mrs K. described the results as nearly miraculous, 'like a ray of light'. Mr K. regained his ability to speak a few words ('he was suddenly able to speak, even if not coherently'), he was able to smile, and he began to wander again. In addition, he again became 'quite agitated and somewhat aggressive', as well as sleepless at night. Mrs K. and her neurologist decided to lower the dosage in the hope that his behavioral problems would cease while his symptomatic gains would continue.

Case 2: Comment

In this case, Mr and Mrs K. are reliving behavioral difficulties, for better or for worse. On the positive side, Mrs K. sees improvement in her husband. On the negative side, Mrs K. is again deeply stressed by her husband's difficult behavior, somewhat fearful, and struggling to find a solution to her new but old problem.

Case 3: 'Get me out of here'

Mrs W. described the case of her mother-in-law, Jenny, who was previously well adjusted to the routine in her nursing home. She was in a relatively benign state emotionally and seemed to be enjoying the art and music programs in which she actively participated. She was described as an 'ideal dementia patient, seemingly happy, content'. Then, after beginning with a new compound, Jenny regained insight into her situation. For example, she remembered that she did not want to be in a nursing home, and she insisted that she be allowed to leave. She also refused to participate in any support programs because the participants are 'too slow for me.'

Case 3: Comment

Jenny might be described as a 'poster child' AD patient, no longer anxious about her losses, and reasonably happy living more or less in the pure present. After a successful early period in a nursing home, she is now noncompliant and resentful of her circumstances. This is disruptive for both Jenny, her family, and the nursing home. If she is allowed to leave, some months later she will reach the same level of incapacitation that justified her nursing home placement to begin with.

Ethical recommendation

New anti-dementia compounds should not be prescribed without special attention to individual cases when patients have already adjusted to their condition, usually in the moderate stage.

Amid the ravages of AD, families and clinicians are easily enchanted and awed by newly approved compounds. For family members there is the potential of regaining the presence of a loved one able to recognize them again and to function better for at least some period of time. For physicians, there is the sense of at least some limited medicinal power over a progressive and incurable disease.

But each patient's response must be carefully monitored with regard to quality of life. Every caregiver should know that the application of a compound is a deeply personal and value-laden decision requiring the careful exercise of compassion and good judgment. Caregivers should know that there is nothing wrong with withdrawing an anti-dementia treatment that does not seem to be enhancing quality of life and of lives. Modest improvement or temporary stabilization of cognitive decline will be viewed by some caregivers as gratifying, but certainly not by all.

Where is the end-point for discontinuing treatment?

How long into the progression of AD should anti-dementia compounds be applied? At some threshold of decline, the level of fragmentation reaches a point where the application of an anti-dementia compound has nothing of benefit to offer (unless the compound contributes, in ways that existing psychiatric medications do not, to the management of behavioral problems in the severe stage). A compound may be recommended for the mild and moderate stages of AD, after which the compound should be withdrawn. We have little knowledge yet of what the experience of patients is upon

withdrawal. This is partly because in many cases families will continue applying the compound beyond the moderate-stage cut-off.

As one group of British observers said:

> No scientific data exist on the effects of stopping treatment with a cholinesterase inhibitor. Patients who took part in the clinical trials continued to take the active drugs with no defined end point. Without controlled data on long term treatment and treatment discontinuation, the decision to stop the drug may be clinically and ethically difficult to make.[4]

There is likely to be a tendency on the part of physicians to continue application of the compound beyond specifications.

The protraction of morbidity

With cholinesterase inhibitors, the underlying neuronal loss is not slowed. This at least precludes the possibility of actually extending the lives of people with AD. Surely no reasonable person would consider such extension of life in the ravages of advanced AD to be a moral or medical goal. In Jonathan Swift's classic *Gulliver's Travels*,

Gulliver encounters among the Luggnaggians the rare 'Struldbrugs' (or 'Immortals'), born only very rarely and distinguished by a red circular spot on their foreheads. Gulliver cries out in rapture, 'Happy nation where every child hath at least a chance for being immortal!' After waxing eloquent about all he would do with immortality, Gulliver is told that the Struldbrugs, when reaching fourscore years, have 'no remembrance of anything but what they learned and observed in their youth and middle age, and even that is very imperfect.' The least miserable among them are those who 'entirely lose their memories'. Gulliver learns that the Struldbrugs 'are despised and hated by all sorts of people'. He reports that the king of the Luggnaggians encouraged him to 'send a couple of Struldbrugs to my own country, to arm our people against the fear of death'.

Compounds such as selegiline and vitamin E, in contrast to the cholinesterase inhibitors, act by reducing neuronal damage.[5] While data suggest no cognitive benefits, but some functional benefits (e.g. eating, using the toilet, grooming), leading to somewhat lower levels of dependence on caregivers, it also appears that these compounds may in some cases delay death. Thus, these substances are a mixed blessing in the sense that while caregiver dependence may be slightly ameliorated, the patient's lifespan may be somewhat enlarged, resulting in more extended caregiving. Of course, eventually, the patient will become entirely dependent with respect to activities of daily living, and the caregiver will finally have to face this reality.

To prevent, delay, ameliorate symptoms and cure AD are all moral goals; to protract morbidity (as though anyone would want to become Struldbrug-like) is not good.

Patient–caregiver wellbeing and delay in nursing home placement

Of concern are studies suggesting that cholinesterase inhibitors may be justified entirely in terms of economic benefits that result from delay in nursing home placement.[6] This delay in placement is suggested as a major benefit in the selegiline and vitamin E study already cited.[5] But surely, delaying institutionalization is an ambiguous goal. In countries where families pay to support nursing home care, delay may mean some saved money; but delay also means that even more burden will be shifted to family caregivers. In countries where long-term care is largely an entitlement, governments will want to keep people with AD in the home if that means less expenditure of tax dollars.

By stating that delay in placement is an aim, we convey to caregivers that, even when they are exhausted and beyond their capacities for caring, there is something wrong (unjust) with placing a loved one in a nursing home.

Further, the aim of delaying placement suggests application of these various compounds throughout the course of AD, or at least until the time of nursing home entrance. This amounts to a virtually permanent application, contrary to what may benefit either the demented patient or caregiver. As indicated in the second section of this chapter, the application of new compounds should be individualized and based on quality of patient life, rather than categorical and routine. A concern with establishing end-points and with the protraction of morbidity was also indicated. The simple-minded application of compounds throughout the course of AD simply for reasons of cost saving seems morally questionable.

Conclusions

As many new anti-dementia compounds are approved in future years, families and society will face remarkably complex ethical issues concerning their proper application, consistent with the principles of autonomy, beneficence, and justice. It is somewhat premature to address this issue without much more extensive outcome data. Yet there is much to be said for anticipating moral quandaries and beginning to establish some frameworks for discussion.

References

1. Rogers SL, Friedhoff LT. The Donepezil Study Group. The efficacy and safety of donepezil in patients with Alzheimer's disease: results of a US multicentre, randomized, double-blind, placebo-controlled trial. Dementia 1996;7:293–303.

2. Sacks O. Awakenings. New York: HarperCollins, 1990:53.

3. Post SG. The moral challenge of Alzheimer's disease. Baltimore: The Johns Hopkins University Press, 1995.

4. Kelly CA, Harvey RJ, Cayton H. Drug treatment for Alzheimer's disease raises clinical and ethical problems. Br Med J 1997;314:693–4.

5. Sano M, Ernesto C, Thomas RG, et al. A
controlled trial of selegiline, alpha-tocopherol, or
both as treatment for Alzheimer's disease. N Engl J
Med 1997;336:1217-22.

6. Knopman D, Schneider L, Davis K, et al. Long-
term tacrine (Cognex) treatment: effects on nursing
home placement and mortality. Neurology
1996;47:166-7.

The family and drug treatments for Alzheimer's disease

Henry Brodaty

10

Alzheimer's disease (AD) is more than one person's illness. It affects patients, families and more extended kin. Conversely, the family has an important influence on the patient and the disease. AD is a disease that has profound social and economic consequences for the wider community. The advent of drug treatments for AD heralds a significant change in the management of this condition.

Families are the most important element in AD management. Their hopes, aspirations and desperation will influence treatment and outcome. The incursions of AD inexorably alter the homeostasis of the patient–caregiver (CG) relationship, which will continue to be changed by the disease's progression and, potentially, further by responsiveness to drug treatment. An understanding of the interaction of the disease, the patient and the family is therefore crucial in maximizing the potential benefits of drug treatments for AD.

This chapter will focus on the role of the family in the drug treatment of AD, and the effects of treatment on the family.

The family, the patient and the disease

Psychological effects of AD on patients

Forgetfulness associated with aging is accepted as inevitable. However, increasing memory loss and failure of other cognitive functions may leave affected persons with feelings of frustration, perplexity, anxiety and depression. Suspicious that a sinister process is enveloping them, persons with early dementia are less likely than their spouses or other family members to seek a diagnosis. Once a diagnosis is made, the person—now a patient—is likely to experience the reactions outlined earlier, as well as grief, disbelief, denial and anger.

Patients with dementia have higher than expected rates and levels of depression. This may be a reaction to knowing that they have this diagnosis or may be inherent in the disease process itself.[1] Other behavioural and psychological signs and symptoms of dementia (BPSSD), such as aggression, agitation,

wandering and psychosis, tend to occur more commonly in the middle and later stages of the disease, complicating its management and causing considerable distress to caregivers.[2-5]

Effects of AD on caregivers

Research on dementia caregivers (CGs) has burgeoned over the past two decades and attests to the high level of psychological distress experienced as well as the high level and rate of depression compared to age- and sex-matched control populations. Scores on general measures of psychological morbidity such as the General Health Questionnaire (GHQ)[6] or specific measures of depression such as the Beck Depression Inventory (BDI)[7] and rates of depression using standardized diagnostic criteria (DSM-III[8], DSM-III-R[9]) are consistently high.[10-12]

Certain stages in the course of the dementia appear to be particularly distressing to CGs: at diagnosis, when the patient loses a key ability, when behavioural complications occur, at the point of institutionalization and at death. Turning to the first of these, the news of a diagnosis of AD is akin to being told that the loved one has cancer. Family members may react

Table 10.1
Model demonstrating factors leading to development of caregiver strain.

Exacerbating factors	Dementia	Protective factors
Social isolation	Dependency and	Practical support
Lack of knowledge	problem behaviours	Family help
Poor skills	↓	Problem-focused coping
Immature coping	Burden on caregiver	
Guilt	↓	
Poor marital relationship	Caregiver strain	
High expressed emotion	Psychological	
Behavioural disturbances	Physical	
Secondary role strain	Financial	
	Social	

with disbelief, anger, resignation or a flurry of activity designed to prove the pronouncement incorrect. These 'hyperactive' families often seek multiple medical opinions and then pursue all manner of treatments, including alternative, unconventional and even fraudulent ones. These may be the CGs who are most vigorous in their insistence that drug treatments be provided and are most unrealistic in their expectations of treatment effectiveness.

A useful model of the effects of dementia on CGs, adapted from that of Poulshock and Deimling,[13] is shown in Table 10.1. Dementia is associated with decline in the patient's abilities, increasing dependence on the CG and the development of BPSSD. These represent an *objective burden* or *stress* on the family CG. Caregivers vary in their capacity to cope, how they react and the *subjective burden* or *strain* that they experience. For some CGs the onset of urinary incontinence may be devastating, whereas others cope without obvious distress. The strain that CGs experience may be manifested psychologically (as outlined previously), physically (with poor physical health and increased use of health services), socially (with increasing social isolation) and financially.

Many variables can amplify CG strain. First, patient variables such as the degree of deterioration, the lack of communicativeness, personality changes and the development of BPSSD have been associated with more CG strain.[4,10] Second, CG variables, such as immature coping skills, poor physical health and poor psychological health, are associated with greater strain. Third, the nature of the relationship between the CG and patient influences the degree of distress that the CG experiences. Thus, more psychological stress is evident in spouses than in children, in wives than in husbands, in CGs who cohabitate than in those who manage from a distance, in care providers than in care managers, and in CGs who have previously had a poor relationship with the patient.[14] On the other hand, the wider family, neighbourhood and social network may exert a beneficial influence, with informal support, i.e. that from family and friends, especially able to ameliorate the adverse effects of caregiving.

Caregiver distress warrants intervention not only to reduce CG suffering, but also because it has importance as a mediator in the progression of the course of AD. Caregiver distress is a powerful predictor of institutionalization of the patient and may even influence patient mortality.[15,16] Moreover, there is some evidence linking CG and patient psychological morbidity, suggesting that attention to the psychological state of the CG may have positive repercussions on the patient.[17]

The consequences of introducing drug treatments into this complex pattern of interactions are largely unexplored. Clearly, if the drugs are able to emend, halt or abate the disease progression this will have powerful effects on family CGs. Furthermore, there may be non-specific results from taking pharmaceutical treatments. These are discussed below.

Hope concerning drug treatments

Unrealistic expectations

Regular and frequent stories in the media, usually sensationalized, fuel public expectations about the latest breakthrough in drug treatments. There may be stories of previously demented Nobel Prize laureates returning to the laboratory after taking tacrine, or the latest report on vitamin or antioxidant research. Families, and to a lesser extent people with dementia, are desperate and will grasp at straws if they perceive there to be even an outside chance of help. Many families feel that they must do something; any form of activism is considered preferable to passive waiting. Others, particularly in non-Western and non-industrial societies, have no expectations of treatment and fatalistically accept their lot.

Families who decide to instigate drug treatment face a bewildering array of alternatives. There are now scores of drugs under clinical trial, of which at least two—tacrine and donepezil—have received licensing approval widely. Word of mouth, media reports, and, for some, careful analysis of competing claims, may influence CGs and patients in their decision on whether to embark on drug treatment and if so, which regimen to use. More often, patients and families rely on their doctors to advise them on the best alternatives.

Many families and patients have unrealistic expectations of a cure, reversal or prolonged stabilization of the disease. This lack of insight may reflect a denial of the inevitable decline, for, as yet, treatments cannot halt disease progression, but rather, delay the progression of symptoms. Some patients, and occasionally relatives, are antipathetic to drug treatments, which they fear will prolong a life without joy.

The placebo response

'The placebo is a powerful widespread phenomenon which relieves many conditions ... and which depends on the patient's belief or expectation that the therapy is effective.'[18] Participants in drug trials for AD appear to exhibit a placebo response. Studies of anti-Alzheimer drugs consistently demonstrate less deterioration amongst patients on placebo than expected from naturalistic longitudinal studies. For example, in the 30-week multicentre US trial of tacrine, 40% of AD patients on placebo remained unchanged or improved.[19] In virtually all of the cholinergic drug trials (e.g. donepezil, rivastigmine), subjects on placebo improved in cognitive function in the first few weeks.

The less than expected rate of decline in patients participating in drug trials is of interest. While this may in part result from a selection bias, in that participating subjects are likely to be better educated and more motivated, it may also result from the expectations of patients and their carers. Albert et al[20] evaluated whether participation in clinical trials affects long-term outcome in AD. Of 215 subjects enrolled in prospective studies of outcomes in AD, 101 participated in randomized clinical trials during the first 2 years of follow-up. These subjects were followed up for 3.5 years and compared with subjects who met eligibility requirements for randomized controlled trials but did not participate ($N = 57$) and with subjects who were ineligible ($N = 57$). Mortality, risk of hospitalization and onset of severe functional deficits did not differ between the groups but the risk of nursing home admission was significantly lower ($P = 0.01$) among trial participants (16.8%) compared with eligible non-participants (36.8%) and ineligible subjects (31.6%). The authors pointed out that the difference in risk of nursing home placement may have represented a long-term benefit of the drug to patients, a selection effect, or a positive effect on CGs in that greater contact with a medical service may have been associated with better caregiving outcomes.

The benefits of placebo are apparent in settings other than randomized clinical trials. For many years, KH3 has been one of the most popular drugs believed to boost cognitive function in the elderly, despite it having no demonstrable efficacy.[21] Faith healing, chelation therapy, chiropracty, natural therapies, herbal medicines and variety of other interventions all have their adherents, despite their lack of proven efficacy as treatments of AD.[22,23] Of course, some of these (e.g. vitamin E[24] and gingko biloba[25,26]) may yet turn out to have demonstrable drug-specific benefits.

The commonest explanation of the placebo effect points to the expectations of the subject. Potential placebo reactors can be identified before a trial by simply asking subjects what they expect to be the outcome.[18] Those who doubt the drug's efficacy do not respond to the placebo, while those with high expectations do.[27] Expectation is also known as belief, faith, confidence, enthusiasm, response bias, transference and anticipation.[28] A desire to believe, please and obey the doctor will increase the effect, while hostility decreases it. Thus, part of the patient expectation will depend on the confidence, enthusiasm and charisma of the therapist.[18] Furthermore, expectations can be (covertly) 'infectious', as patients and their families often talk to each other and reach a consensus. In the cases of dementia this is clearly apparent by observing the interactions of subjects and their CGs in clinic waiting rooms. In our survey of 54 CGs of

subjects about to participate in randomized clinical trials of new drugs for AD,
48% were very hopeful that drugs would
be of benefit, 28% were moderately
hopeful, 22% were somewhat hopeful
and 2% were not at all hopeful (Brodaty
and Luscombe, unpublished observations).

Another explanation of the placebo
effect is that drug treatments may help
to allay the anxieties of patients and
CGs, engender hope and positive
expectations, and lift mood. These
affective changes may influence cognitive performance and account for some
of the benefits seen with placebo.

Involvement with drug treatments, be
they in ordinary clinical practice or as
part of clinical trials, requires patients
and their families to interact more with
medical and other health professionals.
Attention, time, concern, stimulation and
a general feeling of activism ('something
is being done') are all helpful in promoting positive outcomes. There is a general
belief in our community that drugs are
powerful and beneficial, so provision of
any treatment is likely to elicit a conditioned response. The more powerful
the drug and the more powerful the
technique in its administration (intravenous versus intramuscular versus oral),

the more powerful the placebo response
will be. Wall[18] quotes work to demonstrate that even the colour and shape of
oral medication are important: capsules
containing coloured beads are more
effective than coloured tablets, which
are superior to white tablets with
corners, which are better than round,
white tablets. All are inferior to intramuscular saline injections, which in turn are
inferior to intravenous injections.

Finally, an important determinant of
the placebo effect, seen more boldly in
dementia than in other areas of
placebo research, is the interaction
between patient and CG. People with
dementia are increasingly dependent on
their CG for advice as well as basic
care. The well-recognized head-turning
sign, in which the patient turns to his
or her supporter for assistance with the
answer to a question, is an obvious
example of this. Even patients who are
legally competent to give consent,
usually ask the caregiver to decide
about research participation.

Participating in drug trials

The 1990s has witnessed an avalanche
of clinical trials of new drugs for AD.
The role of the family in these drug
trials is critical for a number of reasons.

Recruitment

The motivation for subjects to participate in trials usually comes from the family. Hope and positive expectations, often fuelled by media reports or by word of mouth, are common reasons for enrolment. Often it is the CG who is more motivated to participate than the patient. Sometimes other family members such as children are the driving force. Occasionally, monetary considerations are the motivation, as available drugs may be too expensive to purchase, while trial medications are provided free of charge.

The process of recruitment can be quite stressful on subjects and their families. If the patient satisfies entry criteria there is a feeling of acceptance and success. The corollary is that those rejected feel disappointed, cheated and even angry. Most clinics conducting trials have instituted procedures to deal with this, such as offering alternative trials or treatments.

Sometimes recruitment creates particular difficulties. Patients may for the first time be confronted with their diagnosis, 'Alzheimer's disease', as they read the consent form which must specify the reason why the drug is being precribed. Usually, there is harmonious agreement among the important players in the drug trial—CGs want something done, researchers need subjects for their trials and patients want to get better. Occasionally there is conflict between patient and CG which should lead to a careful re-appraisal as to who is the primary target of the trial. Sometimes, patients are resistant to any intervention which may delay their demise, as they consider themselves to be a burden on their family.

Consent procedures vary from country to country. As a rule, clinical triallists prefer subjects who can give informed consent themselves, though this begs the question of how to ascertain a threshold for legal capacity to give informed consent. Many, but not all, legal authorities also require the family CG to provide written consent. Where trials are expressly designed for the treatment of moderate to late-stage AD, patients are no longer able to give informed consent, which can only be provided by the family CG or by an independent legal authority. Debate continues about the probity of performing research on subjects who cannot give informed consent.[29]

Another area of potential conflict is withdrawal from trials. Consent procedures generally include a statement that subjects can withdraw from a trial at any time without jeopardizing their care from the clinic or treating doctor. Patients and families sometimes have different views about about whether to continue in drug trials. Most drug trial centres would consider it essential to try to resolve these differences with open discussions; otherwise the patient's view prevails.

With an increasing number of drugs available, the competing claims by their manufacturers may create confusion and uncertainty in the minds of subjects and family CGs. General practitioners, community support organizations such as the Alzheimer's Association and specialists not involved in the drug trial can advise patients and CGs about these decisions.

Participation

The family CG has a crucial role once the patient is a participant in the trial. CGs are asked to ensure compliance, monitor the effects and side-effects and, in some trials, rate outcome. Subjects may feel infantilized and scrutinized by this procedure. For example, constant reminders to the patient to take the medication may be seen as overbearing; constant questions about side-effects or checking on compliance can be intrusive and annoying; and ratings of outcome by family CGs can make patients feel like guinea pigs. In the majority of cases such negative reactions do not occur and family CGs handle participation sensitively and in a positive manner.

One university professor in his early 60s was on a trial of a cholinergic agonist which had to be given four times a day. His wife, a few years younger, and extremely active in several organizations, supervised his medication morning and night and rang twice daily to ensure that the midday and 4.00 pm doses were taken as prescribed. The professor was still working in a semi-retired capacity and resented these frequent calls. He found each telephone call a telling and painful reminder of his affliction.

Other persons important in drug trial participation are the extended family and general practitioners. Family members may have different views about participation in drug trials, anti-medical biases, difficulties in accepting the diagnosis of AD or unrealistic expectations of treatment; these can complicate trial participation. Patients and families often turn to their general practitioner for advice, underscoring the need to keep the family doctor informed of the process. Additionally, general practitioners need to be aware of possible side-effects and drug interactions.

Families, drugs and psychodynamics

The ingestion of pills symbolizes internalization of the power of the doctor. This makes patients feel better; it also makes doctors feel good that they have provided something. Indirectly, family CGs may feel that they have contributed to this process by arranging the prescription of drugs. The positive transference between doctor and patient, as well as between doctor and CG, enhances the placebo actions of the drug.

As mentioned earlier, family dynamics alter with progression of dementia, and this can be further influenced by drug treatment. In the past, the patient may have been the more independent and dominant partner, the activist in the family. Gradually, the spouse takes over this role. The inevitable and irretrievable changes in the marital balance may be negative or positive. Administration of pills can be the concrete manifestation of this shift in power. Sometimes the dementing

person, especially if male, resents his partner's good health and bridles at having a 'carer'. Occasionally, relationships improve: a woman who had always been subjugated by a despotic, rigid and somewhat cruel husband found that as his dementia worsened he became more dependent on her, more considerate and affectionate, and less controlling. Her administration of pills to him was gratefully accepted.

Families face considerable dilemmas when dealing with patients who refuse medications, whether they be for medical conditions such as thyroid disease or diabetes, for psychiatric or behavioural complications of dementia, or for the dementia itself. Some families use subterfuge to overcome noncompliance, e.g. representing an anti-psychotic as a vitamin, or surreptitiously concealing the medication in food or liquid. Aside from the ethical issues of such practices, the potential for paranoia and loss of trust need to be considered, although there 'may be some situations where telling lies adheres more to the principle of non-maleficence than respect for autonomy.'[30] Of course, patients who are enrolled in clinical trials and then refuse to take medication must be withdrawn from the study.

Potential benefits and costs to caregivers of drug treatments for dementia

The aim of most drug treatments to date is to delay progression of symptoms and maintain function over time. Evidence of the efficacy of drugs in doing this is provided elsewhere in this book (see Chapters 6 and 8). What remains unclear is the effect on CGs of drug treatments. On the positive side, effective medication can delay loss of independence and thus decrease the amount of time required of CGs in attending to basic functions. In one study, drug treatment with velnacrine significantly improved cognitive function relative to placebo and this was associated (at trend level only) with decreased unpaid caregiving time.[31] Specifically, CGs of patients in the high-dose velnacrine group (225 mg/day) experienced partial release from their time involvement, especially in the area of patient supervision, by an average of 3.3 hours per day. The authors suggested that unpaid CG time demand was directly related to changes in cognitive function and could be useful as an additional outcome measure in clinical trials.

To date, no studies have looked at the effects on CGs' psychological morbidity and sense of wellbeing as a result of specific drug treatments for AD. Preliminary data from our study of CGs of subjects participating in drug trials for AD indicate high levels of psychological morbidity prior to the onset of the trial, with two-thirds of CGs having significant levels of psychological morbidity and a trend for these levels to fall 6 months later (Brodaty and Luscombe, unpublished observations). It is unclear whether these gains are maintained. Paradoxically, long-term use of drugs could even increase CG burden, as there is some evidence that anti-AD drugs may delay institutionalization[32] and even death. It is known that CG stress levels are highest for carers living with patients, high when the patients are in nursing homes and lowest after they have died.[14] Long-term studies of the effects of anti-AD drugs on CGs are warranted.

Drug treatments for AD incur financial and non-financial costs as well. There is the cost of the drug itself, the time taken to obtain, administer and monitor the drug, and the extra medical consultations and investigations. In a study of medication-related stressors among CGs of family members (though not necessarily affected by dementia), medication-related tasks accounted for 7.7% of the total caregiving time. Medications contributed substantially to CGs' stress, with 10 of the 31 CGs interviewed (32%) reporting problems directly related to medications, 6 (19%) reporting problems in managing the drug regimen currently, and 16 (52%) affirming such problems within the past year.[33]

The trajectory of AD is linked closely to increasing dependency of patients on CGs for everyday needs. Estimates of this commitment by CGs to their dementing family members suggest that 80% of CGs provide assistance 7 days a week, and that unemployed wives and husbands spent 116 and 105 hours per week on average, respectively, giving care to their afflicted spouses, while employed wives and husbands spend 58 and 68 hours per week, respectively, in caregiving activities.[34,35] CGs have higher rates of psychological distress,[14] higher rates and levels of clinical depression,[12] and poorer self-rated physical health,[36] but visit their doctors less often than non-CGs.[37,38] CGs' perception of the quality and adequacy of informal support, as opposed to the actual amount of assistance received, also influences emotional health.[14,39]

Despite evidence that memory problems contribute to noncompliance in older persons, only half of CGs

participate in administration of medication.[35] Patients with dementia usually retain the ability to unscrew the caps of bottles and remove tablets, but their abilities to read labels, understand an administration regimen and differentiate medications are limited.[37,40]

Recommendations for CGs to oversee medication have been shown to result in high compliance.[41] CGs appear reasonably knowledgeable about the prescription medications which they are administering. In one study, 92% of CGs could identify the indication for the medication but only 13% could identify the major adverse effects.[42] On the other hand, 62% of patients/CGs attending a psychogeriatric clinic were inaccurate in reporting the patient's current medication, but so were 62% of clinic doctors and 70% of general practitioners when compared to the actual drug inventory established by home visit.[43]

Practical guidelines for management of medications by CGs have been proposed.[35] The use of calendars, pill counts, dosette boxes, Webster packs, and liquid medications if swallowing problems occur, may assist. CGs need instruction on the likely benefits and side-effects, and how to monitor patients for these.

The family and symptomatic treatments for behavioural and psychological signs and symptoms of dementia (BPSSD)

Behavioural and psychological signs and symptoms are common in dementia. Delusions or paranoid ideation occur in a third of patients with AD at some time during the course of their dementia, hallucinations in a sixth and misidentification symptoms in a third.[2,3,44] Rates of major depression of up to 86% have been reported for major depression in patients with dementia, though modal rates are of the order of 20%, and more recent studies suggest more conservative, but nevertheless higher than expected, rates of 5–10%.[1] Aggression, wandering, insomnia, personality clashes and socially inappropriate behaviour are some of the other frequent complications of dementia.[45]

There is robust evidence that BPSSD are the most important contributors to psychological distress in family CGs, accounting for approximately 25% of the variance in morbidity, strain or stress scores.[16] Further, they are important predictors of institutionalization and may portend more rapid decline and earlier death.[46]

Strategies that can prevent, alleviate or reverse the occurrence of BPSSD can provide major benefits to family CGs as well as to patients. Prevention and behavioural interventions are the first line of management for BPSSD. When these fail, drugs may be indicated.

Family CGs may be involved in administering the drugs and monitoring their effects as outlined above. The limited efficacy of psychotropics for BPSSD, the delay in the onset of benefit and the occurrence of side-effects may be distressing to CGs. Careful explanation of the benefits and risks of medication beforehand are important. Also, forewarning CGs of the trial and error nature of many pharmacological treatments of BPSSD may reduce their frustration.

Recommendations

When using drugs in the treatment of patients with AD, the following recommendations may be helpful.

Realistic expectations

Both patients and families require education about what to expect from the drugs: what the potential beneficial effects and side-effects are, and how to monitor efficacy.

Clear instructions

Family CGs need clear instructions on the indications for the medication, method of administration (how to take it, when to take it), contact telephone numbers—including emergency telephone—in case of questions, and possible drug interactions.

Liaison

Liaison with other doctors and health professionals involved in the care of the patient is crucial. This is especially important with the family's general practitioner, to whom CGs will often turn for advice. It may be useful to run educational programs for general practitioners.

Awareness

Awareness in the community about drugs for AD and current trials can assist with recruitment. Accurately portrayed information about trials can dispel unrealistic expectations. Liaison with Alzheimer's associations is helpful.

Other medications

An important principle in reducing the stress associated with administration of medication is to minimize the number of tablets and the frequency with

which they must be taken. Checking for potential drug interactions is vital.

Comprehensive plan of management

Family CGs should be aware that pharmacotherapy is not the only, or even the main, component of management. The contribution of the CG should be acknowledged and supported. Researchers designing future drugs trials for AD might consider factorial designs to test the interaction of drug treatments and family CG interventions. Assessment of the effects on CGs as a secondary outcome measure should be considered in future dementia drug trials.

Supervision

Regular support of patients and family CGs, continued supervision of drugs and frequent medical reviews are required. Family CGs should be informed that symptomatic drug treatments, e.g. anti-psychotics or anti-depressants for BPSSD, can often be withdrawn after a period of time.

Rights of participants in research

The rights of participants in research should be respected, namely: that the research is carried out in a manner conforming with internationally recognized principles; that participants are fully informed and comprehend all the procedures involved in the research and possible associated risks, discomforts from side-effects and inconveniences; that participants have all identifying information about them kept confidential unless they have agreed otherwise; and that consent is voluntary and can be withdrawn at any time without jeopardy to future treatment from that doctor or hospital.

Informed consent

Informed consent should be received before prescribing medication. Where patients are unable to do this the family CG is usually the most appropriate person to do so (depending on local legislation) and assumes responsibilities similar to that of a parent giving permission for a child to receive medication.

In some jurisdictions, guardians must be appointed to approve drugs for those who are incapable of giving informed consent. Legal procedures for participation in research trials are complex and varied.[29]

Conclusion

It is naive to conceptualize recommending drugs for any condition as merely writing a prescription. While medications are playing an increasing role in the management of the dementias, it is not just the patient and doctor who are centre stage. The family CG is a key player who must be consulted throughout the management of this condition.

Acknowledgments

My thanks go to Georgina Luscombe, Wendy Gray, Brian Draper and Kerrie Eyers for their help.

References

1. Brodaty H, Luscombe GI. Depression in patients with dementia. Int Psychogeriatrics 1996;8:609–22.

2. Burns A, Jacoby R, Levy R. Psychiatric phenomena in Alzheimer's disease I: disorders of thought content. Br J Psychiatry 1990;157:72–6.

3. Burns A, Jacoby R, Levy R. Psychiatric phenomena in Alzheimer's disease II: disorders of perception. Br J Psychiatry 1990;157:76–81.

4. Gilleard CJ. Living with dementia. London: Croom Helm, 1984.

5. Rubin EH, Drevets WC, Burke WJ. The nature of psychotic symptoms on senile dementia of the Alzheimer type. J Geriatr Psychiatry Neurol 1988;1:16–20.

6. Goldberg PD. The detection of psychiatric illness by questionnaire. London: Oxford University Press, 1972.

7. Beck AT, Ward CH, Mendelson M, Mock J, Erbaugh J. An inventory for measuring depression. Arch Gen Psychiatry 1961;4:53-63.

8. American Psychiatric Association. Diagnostic and statistical manual, 3rd edn. Washington DC: American Psychiatric Press, 1980.

9. American Psychiatric Association. Diagnostic and statistical manual, 3rd edn revised. Washington DC: American Psychiatric Press, 1987.

10. Morris RG, Morris LW, Britton PG. Factors affecting the emotional wellbeing of the caregivers of dementia sufferers. Br J Psychiatry 1988;153:147-56.

11. Gallagher D, Rose J, Rivera P, Lovett S, Thompson LW. Prevalence of depression in family caregivers. Gerontologist 1989;29:449-56.

12. Mittelman MS, Ferris SH, Shulman E, et al. A comprehensive support program: effect on depression in spouse-caregivers of AD patients. Gerontologist 1995;35:792-802.

13. Poulshock SW, Deimling GT. Families caring for elders in residence: issues in the measurement of burden. J Gerontol 1984;39:230-9.

14. Brodaty H, Hadzi-Pavlovic D. Psychosocial effects on carers of living with dementia. Aust NZ J Psychiatry 1990;24:351-61.

15. Brodaty H, McGilchrist C, Harris L, Peters K. Time until institutionalization and death in dementia patients: role of caregiver training and risk factors. Arch Neurol 1993;50:643-50.

16. Brodaty H. Caregivers and behavioural disturbances: effects and interventions. Int Psychogeriatrics 1996;8:455-8.

17. Brodaty H, Luscombe G. Psychological morbidity in caregivers is associated with depression in patients with dementia. Alzheimers Dis Assoc Disord 1998 (in press).

18. Wall TD. Pain and the placebo response in experimental and theoretical studies of consciousness. Ciba Found Symp 1993;174:187-216.

19. Knapp MJ, Knopman DS, Solomon PR, Pendlebury WW, Davis CS, Gracon SI. A 30-week randomized controlled trial of high-dose tacrine in patients with Alzheimer's disease. JAMA 1994;271:985-91.

20. Albert SM, Sano M, Marder K, et al. Participation in clinical trials and long term outcomes in Alzheimer's disease. Neurology 1997;49:38-43.

21. Brodaty H, Rejuvenation with KH3: fact or fantasy? Curr Therapeut 1989;May:15-23.

22. Coleman LM, Fowler LL, Williams ME. Use of unproven therapies by people with AD. J Am Geriatr Soc 1995;43:747-50.

23. Gurwitz AH. Editorial, Unconventional medicine and AD. J Am Geriatr Soc 1995;43:829-30.

24. Sano M, Ernesto C, Thomas RG, et al. A two-year, double-blind randomized multicenter trial of selegiline and α-tocopherol in the treatment of Alzheimer's disease. N Engl J Med 1997;336:1216-22.

25. Haase J, Halama P, Horr R. Effectiveness of brief infusions with gingko biloba special extract Egb 761 in dementia of the vascular and Alzheimer type. Z Gerontol Geriatr 1996;29:302-9.

26. Lebars PL, Katz MM, Berman N, Itil TM, Freeman AM, Schatzberg AF. A placebo-controlled, double-blind, randomized trial of an extract of gingko biloba for dementia. JAMA 1997;16:1327-32.

27. Bootzin RR. The role of expectancy in behaviour change. In: White LP, Tursky B, Schwartz GE, eds. Placebo: theory, research and mechanisms. New York; Gilford Press, 1985:121-34.

28. Turner JL, Gallimore R, Fox-Henning C. An annotated bibliography of placebo research. J Suppl Abstr Serv Am Psychol Assoc 1980;10:22.

29. Dresser R. Mentally disabled research subjects: the enduring policy issues. JAMA 1996;276:67-72.

30. Cutcliffe J, Milton J. In defence of telling lies to cognitively impaired elderly patients. Int J Geriatr Psychiatry 1996;11:1117-18.

31. Clipp EC, Moore MJ. Caregivers time use: an outcome measure in clinical trial research on Alzheimer's disease. Clin Pharmacol Ther 1995;58:228-36.

32. Knopman D, Schneider L, Davis K, et al. Long-term tacrine (Cognex) treatment: effects on nursing home placement and mortality. Tacrine Study Group. Neurology 1996;47:155-77.

33. Ranelli PL, Aversa SL. Medication-related stressors among family caregivers. Am J Hosp Pharm 1994;51:75-9.

34. Select Committee on Aging, House of Representatives. Exploding the myths: caregiving in America (Publication No. 99-611). Washington DC: US Government Printing Office, 1987.

35. White W, Clipp EC, Hanlon JT, Schmader K. The role of the caregiver in the drug treatment of dementia. CNS Drugs 1995;4:58-67.

36. Schulz R, Vistainer P, Williamson GM. Psychiatric and physical morbidity effects on caregiving. J Gerontol 1990;45:181-91.

37. Wright LK, Clipp EC, George LK. Health consequences of caregiver stress. Med Exerc Nutr Health 1993;2:181-95.

38. Baumgarten M, Hanley JA, Infante-Rivard C, Battista RN, Becker R, Gauthier S. Health of family members caring for elderly persons with dementia: a longitudinal study. Ann Intern Med 1994;120:126-32.

39. George LK, Gwyther LP. Caregiver well-being: a multidimensional examination of family caregivers of demented adults. Gerontologist 1986;26:253-9.

40. Meyer ME, Schuna AA. Assessment of geriatric patients' functional ability to take medication. Drug Intell Clin Pharm 1989;23:171-4.

41. Weinberger M, Samsa GP, Smader K, Greenberg SM, Carr DB, Wildman DS. Compliance with the recommendations from an outpatient geriatric consultation team. J Appl Gerontol 1994;13:455-67.

42. Mallet L, King T. Evaluating family caregivers' knowledge of medication. J Geriatr Drug Ther 1993;7:47-58.

43. Anderson DN, Prunty N, Partridge M, Sexton J. Does anyone know what medication the patient should be taking? Int J Geriatr Psychiatry 1994;9:573-6.

44. Wragg RE, Jeste DV. Overview of depression and psychosis in Alzheimer's disease. Am J Psychiatry 1989;147:577-87.

45. Carrier L, Brodaty H. Mood and behaviour management. In: Gauthier S, ed. Clinical diagnosis and management of Alzheimer's disease. London: Martin Dunitz Ltd, 1996:205-20

46. Steele C, Rovner B, Chase GA, Fostein M. Psychiatric symptoms and nursing home placement of patients with Alzheimer's disease. Am J Psychiatry 1990;145:1049-51.

Steps toward optimal use of Alzheimer-specific drugs

Sanford I Finkel

Accurate diagnosis

Any concerns about cognitive decline in an older person should result in an initial assessment to rule out dementia. It is critical to make the diagnosis as early as possible to address issues of future planning such as financial, legal or driving concerns. It also provides the opportunity to introduce treatment that may slow the decline of the illness and to avoid additional diagnostic or therapeutic tests for other illnesses. Often, family members may be in denial and may not want to hear that their loved one is afflicted with dementia, or they may not understand the nature of the illness, and physicians may hesitate to tell them, not wanting to upset them. Nevertheless a thorough history must be obtained from the patient, as well as a reliable caregiver, with particular emphasis on an established previous baseline of functioning. It is important to determine how long the symptoms have been present, the family history, and the past and present medical psychiatric history. Treatable causes of cognitive decline, especially delirium, must be diagnosed, ruled out, or treated. Between 5% and 15% of patients with symptoms compatible with dementia have a reversible cognitive impairment, most likely related to medications, the presence of depression, or alcohol abuse.[1] The Mini Mental State Examination (MMSE)[2] acts as a good screen for a range of cognitive functions, but may be normal in highly educated people with Alzheimer's disease or abnormally low in non-demented individuals with poor education or those from different cultures. Some clinicians use a relatively brief neuropsychological battery which includes the Benton Temporal Orientation Test[3] and the Hopkins Verbal Learning Test for Recall Learning and Recognition,[4] combined with the Geriatric Depression Scale[5] to rule out depression contributing to cognitive impairment.

Alzheimer's disease (AD) should be viewed as a chronic illness requiring long-term care. The types of cognitive deficits, as well as the behavioral and psychological symptoms, change over time and a variety of pharmacologic and nonpharmacologic treatment alternatives are available. However, the insidious nature of onset and the protracted and steady decline in a wide range of cognitive abilities are characteristic of AD (DSM-IV diagnostic criteria; see Table 11.1).

To make a diagnosis of dementia associated with Lewy body, the patient must be demonstrated to have, in addition to dementia, one of the following three symptoms: detailed visual hallucinations, alterations of alertness or attention, or Parkinsonian signs.[6]

Vascular dementia (VaD) is characterized by a sudden onset of dysfunction in one or more cognitive domains with a stepwise deteriorating course. Often, focal neurologic signs are apparent, such as exaggerated deep tendon reflexes, extensor plantar response, and gait abnormalities. Depression and psychosis are also common complications of VaD. Frequently, there is a history of previous strokes or transient ischemic attacks, as well as risk factors for strokes (coronary artery disease, atrial fibrillation, hypertension).[7]

Neuroimaging techniques have improved diagnostic accuracy. The CT scan is of significance in excluding non-AD dementias. However, AD and VaD may coexist in 10% of all

Table 11.1
Diagnostic criteria for dementia of the Alzheimer's type.

A. The development of multiple cognitive deficits manifested by both:
  (1) memory impairment (impaired ability to learn new information or to recall previously learned information)
  (2) one (or more) of the following cognitive disturbances:
    (a) aphasia (language disturbance)
    (b) apraxia (impaired ability to carry out motor activities despite intact motor function)
    (c) agnosia (failure to recognize or identify objects despite intact sensory function)
    (d) disturbance in executive functioning (i.e. planning, organizing, sequencing, abstracting)
B. The cognitive deficits in criteria A1 and A2 each cause significant impairment in social or occupational functioning and represent a significant decline from a previous level of functioning
C. The course is characterized by gradual onset and continuing cognitive decline.
D. The cognitive deficits in criteria A1 and A2 are not due to any of the following:
  (1) other central nervous system conditions that cause progressive deficits in memory and cognition (e.g. cerebrovascular disease, Parkinson's disease, Huntington's disease, subdural hematoma, normal-pressure hydrocephalus, brain tumor)
  (2) systemic conditions that are known to cause dementia (e.g. hypothyroidism, vitamin B_{12} or folic acid deficiency, niacin deficiency, hypercalcaemia, neurosyphilis, HIV infection)
  (3) substance-induced conditons
E. The deficits do not occur exclusively during the course of a delirium
F. The disturbance is not better accounted for by another axis I disorder (e.g. major depressive disorder, schizophrenia)

From the *Diagnostic and Statistical Manual of Mental Disorders*, 4th edn. (American Psychiatric Association: Washington DC, 1994) 142–3. Used with permission.

demented patients, thus complicating the differentiation between the two.

The physical examination is important to rule out other neurologic or systemic illness. Issues of comorbidity must be considered. Medications and concomitant medical and psychiatric illness contribute to cognitive impairment. A comprehensive laboratory evaluation is necessary to rule out other non-Alzheimer's causes of dementia. This would routinely include a complete blood count, blood chemistries, vitamin B_{12}, thyrotropin stimulating hormone (TSH), serologic test for syphilis, non-contrast head CT or MRI, and other tests as clinically indicated.[8] Promising additional tests which are not currently recommended for routine use include apolipoprotein E and genotype[9], cerebrospinal fluid (CSF), tau-[10] and beta-amyloid[11] proteins.

In almost 88% of patients, the diagnosis of AD can be established based on a general medical evaluation, although neuropsychological testing can aid in confirming an early diagnosis, especially in highly educated individuals.

The NINCDS–ADRDA DSM-IV diagnoses sometimes do not fit patients who are in the very early stages of AD. These patients may have one or two cognitive deficits, but do not fulfill all of the diagnostic criteria. There is a need to provide practical guidelines, particularly to primary care physicians, who may not have the time or expertise to conduct a complete history. Further, it is important to arrive at a transnational, cross-cultural consensus as to which questions are most important to ask in a primary care interview. Disease management protocols and decision trees would also be helpful to primary care physicians in arriving at accurate diagnoses and/or need for referral.

Besides cognitive functioning, it is of critical importance to evaluate instrumental activities of daily living, such as ability to use the telephone, manage financial affairs, manage and comply with medication regimens, and utilize transportation. Caregiver input will be of particular importance in assessing functional improvement on pharmacotherapy.

Clinical trials have focused primarily on mild to moderate AD, though there is some evidence to suggest that people with more severe illness may actually demonstrate improvement on AD-specific drugs.

AD has a natural course ranging from 5 to 15 years, and it is not yet clear whether mild, moderate, or severely affected patients improve most with cognitive-enhancing medication. In any therapeutic relationship involving pharmacotherapy, it is also important to provide emotional support for both patients and caregivers. Families must be educated as to the basic facts of AD, the symptoms they can anticipate at different stages of the illness, and environmental changes which can maximize functioning.

To date, pharmacologic treatment for the cognitive deficits of AD has been limited to the cholinesterase inhibitors tacrine and donepezil, which have demonstrated efficacy in mild to moderate stages. There is currently a paucity of information on long-term treatment and on the latter stages of AD with these agents. We will review some of the available data and summarize what we have learned towards optimal use of these drugs. The goal of being to restore cognitive abilities, prevent further decline, and increase functional status.

Tacrine

Tacrine represented a major breakthrough after many unsuccessful attempts to develop effective pharmacotherapy for AD. Although tacrine provides only modest benefits in patients with AD and is associated with adverse events in almost half the patients treated, it has set a precedent

in the field, thus paving the way for other medications with the potential for greater efficacy and tolerance.

Over 2000 patients have been studied in five double-blind, placebo-controlled trials summarized by Schneider and Forette.[12] Overall, 30–40% demonstrated improvement, compared to 10% of those taking placebo. Patients who can tolerate 120–160 mg/day do best, but the benefits beyond 30 weeks are not well known.

Ten to twenty per cent of patients develop cholinergic side-effects. Those taking NSAIDs are most susceptible to nausea and vomiting. Cholinergic effects generally diminish within a few days. Thus, the challenge is to help the patient through the early days of therapy. This may include dropping the dose and re-challenging. Special care must be taken for those patients with bradycardia and concomitant cardiac conduction problems. Thirty per cent of patients on tacrine develop reversible and asymptomatic elevation in liver enzymes (three times the upper limit of normal), and between 5% and 10% need to have medication discontinued because of elevations of 10 times the upper limit of normal or above. However, 80% of those with elevated liver enzyme levels can be successfully treated following discontinuation and reintroduction of tacrine with a slowly increasing dose level.[13]

There is preliminary evidence that the behavioral and psychological symptoms of AD may be reduced by tacrine. Agitation, aberrant motor behaviors, and hallucinations may be reduced for patients on tacrine, regardless of cognitive response. Patients with Lewy body dementia may be particularly responsive to cholinergic treatment.

Tacrine's duration of action is under 7 hours and, thus, multiple daily doses are necessary. Typically, the starting dose is 10 mg, four times a day, with an increase of 10 mg four times a day every six weeks up to a maximum of 40 mg four times a day.

There are reports of changes in hematologic parameters, as well as elevated bilirubin levels. Therefore, some clinicians obtain periodic complete blood counts (CBCs) and full liver profiles.

Tacrine is contraindicated in patients with abnormal transaminase levels, with clinical jaundice with total bilirubin exceeding 3.0 mg/dl, with a history of liver disease, with a history of hypersensitivity to tacrine or an acridine derivative, with a history of strokes, with central nervous system (CNS) tumors, and with those who are unable to eliminate alcohol, given the potential heptatotoxicity of tacrine.

The increase in cognitive functioning in patients taking tacrine is often subtle. It may not be demonstrated by the MMSE. However, the ADAS-Cog subscale is very sensitive to neuropsychological changes and could be administered periodically. Some clinicians recommend that it should be administered 12 weeks and 24 weeks after starting the medication.[14] It is not unusual for an ADAS-Cog to improve 6 points, whereas the MMSE and functional status remain the same, and the physician or caregivers observe no clinical change.

Patients who are on medications with significant anticholinergic effects should generally not take tacrine. Simultaneous administration of tacrine and theophylline may result in an increase in theophylline levels. Ott[15] described a 67-year-old patient with both AD and mild

Parkinson's disease who developed gait abnormalities, severe tremor, and stiffness of extremities on 80 mg of tacrine per day. Levodopa–carbidopa 100/25 mg four times a day produced significant improvement. Thus, patients with both illnesses may benefit from a combination of levodopa–carbidopa and tacrine.

Case 1

Mrs E, an 83-year-old Caucasian female, diagnosed with AD in January 1992, participated in a 16-week, open-label safety study if tacrine in February 1995. Mrs E had previously participated in a clinical trial designed to treat the behavioural symptoms of AD. At screening, Mrs E had moderate AD and was incontinent. Her incontinence was of concern to her caregivers, as was her wandering. The patient also spent much of her time singing loudly and occasionally exclaiming 'This is my son, isn't he wonderful?' Her medical history included diet-controlled diabetes mellitus and medication-controlled hypertension. Mrs E was a non-smoker and had abused alcohol in the past. Her initial dose was 20 mg of tacrine four times a day. This was increased to 30 mg, and then reached the maximum dose of 40 mg four times a day in May. She was maintained on that dose to the end of the trial. She did not experience any gastrointestinal side-effects of the medication, and laboratory tests of liver function remained normal throughout the 16 weeks. Her initial response to the medication included a reversal of her incontinence and a decrease in wandering and agitation. However, from mid-March to the beginning of May, incontinence returned, agitation increased and attention span decreased. Haloperidol (0.5 mg b.i.d.) was prescribed on 25 May 1995 and was administered intermittently by the family. Mrs E completed the study on 5 June 1995 and was put on a regimen of open-label tacrine. Although she continued to wander, incontinence and agitation decreased and her attention span increased slightly. The family felt that tacrine improved the patient's behavior and decided to continue her on tacrine 40 mg four times a day. The patient was able to remain at home, care for by her family, until her death following a hip fracture 18 months later.

Both patients and families should be informed of a limit in improvement, as well as the potential side-effects and financial costs. As of 1996, the daily cost of 160 mg/day of tacrine is approximately $1400 a year. Thirty-two weeks of blood monitoring would cost at least an additional $650. Thus, costs for tacrine exceed $2000 a year. Medicare will cover only the cost of the tacrine monitoring tests. Knopman et al[16] found that patients who responded to tacrine treatment of 80 mg/day or more were less likely to be institutionalized in a nursing home. For those receiving over 120 mg, there was a trend toward lower mortality rates.

Tacrine has been a ground-breaking drug. There are many things to be learned from our experience with tacrine. It should not be discontinued abruptly, because of the risk of psychotic withdrawal symptoms. Further there is tremendous heterogeneity regarding effective doses and adverse events.

Donepezil

Donepezil hydrochloride is a reversible inhibitor of acetylcholinesterase. Administration of food does not significantly affect the rate of extent of donepezil absorption. Donepezil has increasingly replaced tacrine in clinical practice because it causes fewer adverse reactions, and even these are generally mild and short-lived. Donepezil has been studied in patients with MMSEs between 10 and 26 and a clinical dementia rating score of 1 or 2. Hepatotoxicity is not a problem and, thus, one does not need to obtain and monitor ALT levels.

Donepezil is also easier to administer because its long half-life (over 60 h) allows it to be administered on a once-a-day basis. Further, and again in contrast to tacrine, there is almost no titration involved. Patients are prescribed a single 5-mg dose once a day and are re-evaluated after approximately 1 month. For those patients who have demonstrated no improvement, an increase to 10 mg is indicated. Thus, a full therapeutic trial of donepezil can be concluded in less than 3 months, whereas for tacrine, twice the amount of time is necessary.

A 24-week trial of 480 patients on donepezil, 5 or 10 mg a day versus placebo, demonstrated a mean change in ADAS-Cog of 2.49 and 2.88 respectively.[17] Patients who had completed a 14-week placebo-controlled study[18] and who were continued for 2 years on 10 mg/day showed less deterioration than would be expected.[19] Case studies are now being published on patterns of response to donepezil.[20]

Case 2

Mrs EB, and 87-year-old married woman, was referred for evaluation. Her husband of 60 years accompanied her. There was a 3-history of progressive memory loss. The MMSE score was 21. Other causes of dementia were ruled out. She was started on donepezil, 5 mg at night, with no adverse events for the first month of treatment. The MMSE score continued to be 21. At that time, the dose was increased to 10 mg. She experienced nausea and diarrhea, and the dose was temporarily reduced to 5 mg. After 10 days she was re-challenged with 10 mg and had minimal nausea, which disappeared over the next week. The MMSE score improved to 23 by the end of the second month of treatment. Further, her husband indicated that she was playing the piano again and had an easier time dressing herself.

Conclusions

At the time of writing, there are only two approved medications for treating AD in the USA. Donepezil is the first-line treatment because it is at least as efficacious as tacrine, but with no heptatotoxicity and fewer adverse events. Nevertheless, for those previously taking tacrine, and who are benefiting, continued administration is indicated.

Unfortunately, the cholinergic enhancement strategies may improve symptoms or delay the decline caused by the illness for only a short time. Nevertheless, this is a definite benefit for both patient and family. Pharmacology for the cognitive deficits of AD in terms of both cognitive enhancement and delaying decline is in its infancy. The first approved drug, tacrine, has now been followed by donepezil and will be followed by a host of other medications with a range of pharmacokinetic and pharmacodynamic activities. We can state now that the first breakthroughs have occurred, and the future medications promise to be more efficacious, while maintaining high levels of safety and demonstrating minimal adverse events.

References

1. Clarfield AM. Irreversible dementias: do they reverse? Ann Intern Med 1988;109:476–86.

2. Folstein MF, Folstein SE, McHugh PR. Mini Mental State: a practical method for grading the cognitive state of patients for the clinicians. J Psychiatr Res 1975;12:189–98.

3. Benton AL, Hamsher KS, Varney NR, et al. Contributions to neuropsychological assessment. New York: Oxford University Press, 1983.

4. Brandt J. The Hopkins Verbal Learning Test: developed of a new memory test with six equivalent forms. Clin Neuropsychol 1991;5:125–42.

5. Burke WJ, Roccaforte WH, Wengel SP. The short form of the Geriatric Depression Scale: a comparison with the 30-item form. J Geriatr Psychiatry Neurol 1991;4:173-8.

6. McKeith IG, Galasko D, Kosaka K, et al. Consensus guidelines for the clinical and pathological diagnosis of dementia with Lewy bodies (DLB): report of the consortium on DLB international workshop. Neurology 1996;47:1113-14.

7. Rockwood K, Parhad I, Hachinski V, et al. Diagnosis of vascular dementia: Consortium of Canadian Centres for Clinical Cognitive Research Consensus Statement. Can J Neurol Sci 1994;21:358-64.

8. Corey-Bloom J, Thal LJ, Galasko D, et al. Diagnosis and evaluation of dementia. Neurology 1995;45:211-18.

9. National Institute on Aging/Alzheimer's Association Working Group. Apolipoprotein E genotyping in Alzheimer's disease. Lancet 1996;347:1091-5.

10. Galasko D, Clark C, Chang L, et al. Assessment of CSF levels of tau protein in mildly demented patients with Alzheimer's disease. Neurology 1997;48:632-5.

11. Wagner SL, Peskind ER, Nochlin D, et al. Decreased levels of soluble amyloid β-protein precursor are associated with Alzheimer's disease in concordant and discordant monozygous twin pairs. Ann Neurol 1994;36:215-20.

12. Schneider LS, Forette F. AD symptomatic drugs: tacrine. In: Gauthier S, ed. Clinical diagnosis and management of Alzheimer's disease. London: Martin Dunitz Ltd, 1996:221-38.

13. Watkins PB, Zimmerman HJ, Knapp MH, Gracon SI, Lewis KW. Hepatoxic effects of tacrine administration in patients with Alzheimer's disease. JAMA 1994;271:992-8.

14. Woo JK, Lantz MS. Alzheimer's disease: how to give and monitor tacrine therapy. CME Geriatrics 1995;50:50-3.

15. Ott BR, Lannon MC. Exacerbation of parkinsonism by tacrine. Clin Neuropharmacol 1992;15:322-5.

16. Knopman D, Schneider L, Davis K, et al. Long-term tacrine (Cognex) treatment: effects on nursing home placement and mortality. Neurology 1996;47:166-77.

17. Rogers SL, Farlow MR, Mohs R, et al. A 24-week double-blind, placebo-controlled trial of donepezil in patients with Alzheimer's disease. Neurology 1998;50:136-45.

18. Rogers SL, Friedhoff LT, Apter JT, et al. The efficacy and safety of donepezil in patients with Alzheimer's disease: results of a US multicentre, randomized, double-blind, placebo-controlled trial. Dementia 1996;7:293-303.

19. Rogers SR, Friedhoff LT. Long-term efficacy and safety of donepezil in the treatment of Alzheimer's disease: an interim analysis of the results of a US multicentre open label extension study. Eur Neuropsychopharmacol 1998;8:67-75.

20. Mann RJ. Clinical efficacy of donepezil hydrochloride in patients with Alzheimer's disease: case studies. Adv Ther 1997;14:223-33.

Achievements and unresolved issues

Serge Gauthier and Judes Poirier

12

Introduction

In this chapter, general principles of pharmaco-therapy of Alzheimer's disease (AD) will be discussed, primarily based on the experience of the last 12 years using cholinesterase inhibitors (CIs) and selective muscarinic agonists (MAs). Reference will be made to other chapters of this book, where appropriate. We also aim at answering practical questions from clinicians faced with using cholinergic agents in their clinical practice. At this point, (February 1998), three drugs for the control of symptoms of AD have received regulatory approval in some countries (tacrine, donepezil, rivastigmine), and other agents are expected to be approved for general prescription use within a year (metrifonate, propentofylline).

Although there is clearly symptomatic benefit in phase III randomized studies involving probable AD patients, much remains to be learned about the response to treatment in clinical practice with the broader spectrum of patients with possible AD. We will also address the issue of pharmacogenetics, which examines the impact of genetic heterogeneity on clinical responsiveness.

Why is the symptomatic treatment response so modest in AD?

There is certainly a discrepancy between expectations and observed responses from cholinergic agonists: neither CIs nor MAs have demonstrated individually the clinically dramatic symptomatic benefits of L-DOPA in Parkinson's disease (PD), at least in its early stages (so-called 'honeymoon effect'). There may well be physiologic as well as pathologic reasons[1] for the relatively modest symptomatic benefit from cholinergic replacement in AD. Furthermore, brain biopsies have shown that acetylcholine-synthesizing ability as reflected by choline acetyltransferase (CAT) activity is already low in the early stages of AD,[2] and post-mortem studies have demonstrated a severe depletion of CAT activity, particularly in patients carrying the ApoE4 mutation.[3,4]

Another issue is that only monotherapy has been attempted so far in AD. There is indeed a good rationale for combination therapy using agents acting in a synergistic fashion at the cholinergic synapse: a CI should theoretically be combined with a MA, with attention to possibly additive cholinergic side-effects. The pharmacotherapy of PD is again a good model to follow, where combinations of L-DOPA and dopamine agonists have a much stronger clinical impact, as a long-term treatment strategy.

Are we measuring the appropriate outcomes in clinical trials?

The emphasis on cognitive enhancement as the *sine qua non* for an effective AD drug, discussed in Chapter 5, has led to rejection of some promising cholinergic agents which had demonstrated weak effects on the ADAS-Cog, but potentially impressive effect in delaying appearance of neuropsychiatric manifestations of AD, or controlling existing behavioral symptoms.[5] Many clinicians will argue that the non-cognitive effects of cholinergic agents have been understudied, and, if demonstrated in carefully designed monotherapy or combination randomized clinical trials, would have greater acceptance by patients and families, as well as formulary bodies, than a modest cognitive enhancement.

Are we able to measure short-term efficacy in clinical practice?

There is still a debate as to how physicians can assess response to a symptomatic treatment in AD, without the support of nurses, psychometricians and other observers essential to randomized clinical trials in AD. A good baseline prior to treatment is clearly required, establishing cognitive, functional, behavioral and emotional status by interviewing the patient and caregiver, and administering the MMSE and/or other structured questionnaires.[6] Efficacy of and tolerance to treatment are determined by interviewing patient and caregiver, at visits usually set at regular intervals. This strategy, similar to the CIBIC used in clinical trials, can be complemented by structured interviews using the Clinical Dementia Rating[7] domains (memory, orientation, judgment and problem-solving, community affairs, home and hobbies, personal care). A targeted symptom strategy has been proposed,[8] where a shortlist of goals is selected prior to treatment and followed up over time.

Are there long-term symptomatic benefits in AD?

Considering the modest size of effect observed in clinicial trials of 3–6 months' duration for CIs and MAs, it may well be more realistic to extend structured observations to 2 years, even with agents intended to have only symptomatic benefit. The pharmacotherapy of PD is again a good model to follow, where combinations of L-DOPA and dopamine agonists have a much better impact in the long term; a washout of such drugs demonstrates their strictly symptomatic effects, but there is no doubt as to their ability to delay loss of functional autonomy for patients with PD. It is thus proposed to develop strategies for extended observations of treatment benefit in AD, even if the initial response is modest, and establish if there is truly a delay in milestones such as appearance of neuropsychiatric manifestations, loss of functional autonomy and institutionalization. Results from open-labeled tacrine[9]- and donepezil[10]-treated patients are encouraging. Control groups without placebo are a limitation, to be overcome with carefully matched untreated patients.

Can we predict clinical responders?

We can unfortunately predict relatively well which patients will deteriorate faster.[11] We would like very much to be able to predict who will respond to cholinergic therapy. Clinical profiles of responders to CIs are still anecdotal, with reports of enhanced responses in patients with clinical features of Lewy body dementia. We do not yet know if patients with AD and vascular features, parkinsonian features or psychotic features will improve more or less than the typical probable AD patients studied in phase III pivotal studies.

The ApoE genotype is so far the most reliable biological predictor of clinical response: ApoE4 carriers have smaller changes in response to CIs to a great extent because of their severe depletion in CAT.[3] The drugs of choice for them may well be non-cholinergic agents such as Servier 12024, acting by predominantly noradrenergic mechanisms, or propento-fylline, acting by adenosine reuptake, anti-inflammatory and neurotrophic mechanisms. The use of pharmacogenet-ics has been proposed as a strategy to select the best possible treatment for each patient, based on his or her clinical and genetic profile. Preliminary evidence of a gene-dependent drug responsiveness has been obtained for tacrine[3] and Servier S12024.[12] Ongoing randomized clinical trials with tacrine CR, rivastigmine, metri-fonate, SKB202026 and xanomeline will hopefully uncover novel patterns of clini-cal responsiveness based on ApoE

genotype, age, gender, education and family history.

Should we combine cholinergic drugs with stabilization agents?

Although there are few studies that have established a disease stabilization effect using antioxidants such as alpha-tocopherol or monoamine oxidase B inhibitors such as selegiline,[13] it is logical at this time to combine low doses of alpha-tocopherol with a CI. In its final planning stage is a study by the NIA-funded Alzheimer Disease Study Unit to determine if alpha-tocopherol would be a safe and effective means to delay conversion of minimal cognitive impairment to AD. There may also be a potential additive value of estrogens with CIs in postmenopausal women.[14]

When do we start symptomatic therapy for AD?

The currently approved monographs for CIs such as tacrine, donepezil and rivastigmine reflect the populations of patients studies in phase II and III, namely mild to moderate in severity, operationally defined as MMSE scores of 10–26. There are no data currently avail-able from randomized placebo-controlled studies in the later stages of AD, but some are under way, with outcome variables appropriate for disease severity as discussed in Chapter 3.

AD pharmacotherapy can be initiated after confirmation of diagnosis by careful interviews with patient and caregiver, administration of objective tests such as MMSE, documentation of disease pattern on follow-up, treatment of concomitant medical problems such as depression, elimination of non-essential drugs that could interfere with cognition, and discussion about diagnosis and prognosis with patient and caregiver (Table 12.1). The AD drugs should thus never be

Table 12.1
Utilization guidelines for drug treatment in Alzheimer's disease

1. Confirm the diagnosis of dementia (progressive cognitive loss with impact on daily life) by carefully interviewing patient and family/friends and administering an objective test such as the Mini Mental State Examination (MMSE); confirm diagnosis of Alzheimer's disease by documenting a typical pattern of symptoms and progression over time, with unremarkable findings on neurological and physical examination; stage disease severity.
2. Treat concomitant medical problems such as depression, and eliminate nonessential drugs that could interfere with cognition.
3. Discuss diagnosis and prognosis with patient and family; advise on will-making and advance directives while patient's competency is not in doubt; refer to local branch of Alzheimer Society; assess caregiver's health and coping skills.
4. Explain potential effectiveness of Alzheimer-specific medications and the known side-effects.
5. Establish the cognitive, functional, behavioral and emotional status before treatment by interviewing patient and caregiver, and administering MMSE and other structured questionnaires.
6. Start drug therapy following the recommendations from the monograph.
7. Assess efficacy and tolerance to treatment at intervals by interviewing patient and caregiver; maintain dosage if improvement in condition is detected, particularly for functional abilities (ADL, hobbies, social interaction); increase dose if no clear evidence of response and no contraindication.
8. Stop treatment if clinical deterioration is observed despite optimal therapeutic dose or intolerable side-effects.
9. Continue treatment beyond 6 months if there is evidence of functional improvement, disease stabilization or slower decline.
10. Discontinue treatment when disease has progressed to severe stage, in agreement with legal guardian and respecting pre-established advance directives.

prescribed without a careful diagnosis and explanation about the disease. They do not replace, but rather form a part of, a global biopsychological treatment that will span many years.[15]

When do we stop symptomatic therapy for AD?

If there is obvious deterioration of symptoms over 4–6 months despite therapeutic doses of a CI, the drug must be stopped. It should be noted that a cognitive improvement may be associated with a deterioration of mood and behavior, requiring either cessation of the CI or addition of an antidepressant, preferably of the SSRI type.

If there is an obvious improvement in symptoms on a therapeutic dose of a CI, sustained for more than 6 months, there is obviously no reason to discontinue. 'Dramatic' responses can occur in up to 25% of patients, with return to past hobbies or occupations, often with concomitant improvements on the MMSE of 5–6 points. More commonly, the response will be subtle, best described as an increased alertness and interest in family affairs, or an increase in spontaneous speech output. Although difficult to quantify in terms of cost-benefits, these modest effects

can have a profound impact on the family, as discussed in Chapter 10. The duration of treatment must be individualized by continuous dialog with patient and family.

Finally, if there is no observed improvement or deterioration over 6 months at a therapeutic dose, a drug wash-out may be considered to reassess the need for continuation of symptomatic therapy. This issue will be made more complex by the combination of symptomatic and stabilization agents in the near future.

Which drug to use?

Although there are still many data from phase III pivotal studies to be published, and there have been no head-to-head comparisons of different CIs or MAs in one study, we can at this point propose some guidelines to be used in choosing a drug for an individual patient, based on pharmacologic as well as patient characteristics. These guidelines are for cholinergic agents, but will need to be rapidly expanded as non-cholinergic symptomatic drugs and stabilization agents become available. It is our hope that a systematic post-marketing surveillance (PMS) of these agents will give us reliable long-term safety as well as effectiveness data, from which guidelines of utilization can be derived. PMS may also uncover patterns of clinical responses based on clinical profiles such as AD with vascular features, AD with early extrapyramidal features, or AD with early behavioral features, to be confirmed in randomized clinical trials.

As outlined in Chapter 6, the pharmacokinetic and pharmacodynamic properties of the different CIs should be taken into account: acetyl-cholinesterase (AChE) versus butyryl-cholinesterase (BuChE) selectivity, half-lifes of drug in plasma, and reversibility of AChE inhibition. Thus a short-half-life drug such as tacrine requires a four times a day schedule, whereas long-half-life drugs such as donepezil and metrifonate allow a once a day intake. Compliance for persons living alone would obviously be facilitated by a once a day schedule that can be monitored by a phone call or a visit. Since a serious overdose with a CI such as metrifonate having irreversible inhibitory actions on AChE (via its metabolite dichlorvos) may require prolonged monitoring for persistent bradyarrythmias, a limited supply available at a given time may be

preferable. The safety and efficacy profile for a given CI may determine the selection of one drug versus another for different patient groups: if rivastigmine is confirmed based on careful analysis of published data from pivotal studies as having a higher potency than other CIs, albeit with a slightly higher side-effect profile, it may be the drug of choice for young patients with AD, expected to decline more rapidly than older patients. The latter, particularly if frail, female and of low body weight, should be started on the lowest possible dose of the safest CI available.

If there is no therapeutic response to a therapeutic dose of a CI, the current options are to try another CI after an appropriate wash-out (at least 1 month), or to join a randomized clinical trial with a novel agent. Even on placebo treatment there is demonstrable benefit for the patient and family,[16] and, as discussed in Chapter 9, the currently demonstrated efficacy of CIs does not make placebo-controlled studies unethical. If the clinical benefit initially observed with a CI is wearing off, one option is to increase the dose, as tolerated; hopefully, the addition of a MA will soon be possible. The clinical response to CI could be amplified by combination with other agents such as alpha-tocopherol or estrogens (see above), as well as non-pharmacologic approaches such as family intervention[17] and training for preserved cognitive skills.[18]

What is in the pipeline?

As more and more drugs designed to potentiate cholinergic activity are becoming available for general prescription use, the next generation of compounds targeted at disease progression are now entering phases I to III of clinical testing. As examples, estrogens, potent inducers of cholinergic activity, neuronal reinnervation and ApoE levels, are being used in a phase III placebo-controlled randomized study involving female patients with early AD.

In preclinical development, several compounds that inhibit amyloid production or beta-amyloid aggregation, or that promote ApoE synthesis, are currently under study, with phase I clinical testing projected to start within the next 2 years. The full impact of such agents will be felt in later years in their ability to delay onset of AD symptoms in genetically predisposed individuals.

Conclusions

This is a time for optimism in the management of AD, and more specifically in its pharmacotherapy. The investment made over 20 years for a safe and effective cholinergic substitution therapy is coming to fruition, and we can rapidly build on this success with stabilization and preventive approaches. The availability of safe and effective symptomatic drugs for AD is one component of a global biopsychosocial treatment that will span many years, for both the person with AD and his or her caregiver. Whether or not a cholinergic drug has a dramatic or a modest clinical effect for a given patient, the associated care and interest from the health support team will be therapeutic.

References

1. Geula C, Mesulam MM. Cholinergic systems and related neuropathological predilection patterns in Alzheimer disease. In: Terry RD, Katzman R, Bick KL, eds. Alzheimer disease. New York: Raven Press Ltd, 1994:263–91.

2. Gauthier S, Leblanc R, Quirion R, et al. Transmitter-replacement therapy in Alzheimer's disease using intracerebro-ventricular infusions of receptor agonists. Can J Neurol Sci 1986;13:394–402.

3. Poirier J, Delisle MC, Quirion R, et al. Apolipoprotein E4 allele as a predictor of cholinergic deficits and treatment outcome in Alzheimer's disease. Proc Natl Acad Sci USA 1995;92:12260–4.

4. Arendt T, Schindler C, Brickner M, et al. Neuronal remodeling is impaired in patients with Alzheimer's disease carrying apolipoprotein E4 allele. Neuroscience 1997;17:516–29.

5. Bodick NC, Offen WW, Levey AI, et al. Effects of xanomeline, a selective muscarinic receptor agonsit, on cognitive function and behavioral symptoms in Alzheimer's disease. Arch Neurol 1997;54:465–73.

6. Murali Doraiswamy P. Current cholinergic therapy for symptoms of Alzheimer's disease. Primary Psychiatry 1996;3:3–11.

7. Morris JC. The Clinical Dementia Rating (CDR): current version and scoring rules. Neurology 1993;43:2412–14.

8. Rockwood K, Stolee P, Howard K, et al. The use of Global Attainment Scaling in an anti-dementia drug trial. Neuroepidemiology 1996;15:330–8.

9. Knopman D, Schneider L, Davis K, et al. Long-term tacrine (Cognex TM) treatment effects on nursing home placement and mortality. Neurology 1996;47:166–77.

10. Rogers SR, Friedhoff LT. Long-term efficacy and safety of donepezil in the treatment of Alzheimer's disease: an interim analysis of the results of a US multicentre open label extension study. Eur Neuropsychopharmacol 1998;8:67–75.

11. Panisset M, Stern Y. Prognostic factors. In: Gauthier S, ed. Clinical diagnosis and management of Alzheimer's disease. London: Martin Duntiz Publishers, 1996:129–39.

12. Florence R, Helbecque N, Neuman E, et al. ApoE genotyping and response to drug treatment in Alzheimer's disease. Lancet 1997;349:539.

13. Sano M, Ernesto C, Thomas RG, et al. A controlled trial of selegiline, alpha-tocopherol, or both as treatment for Alzheimer's disease. N Engl J Med 1997;336:1216–22.

14. Schneider LS, Farlow MR, Henderson VW, et al. Effects of estrogen replacement therapy on response to tacrine in patients with Alzheimer's disease. Neurology 1996;46:1580–4.

15. Gauthier S, Panisset M, Nalbantoglu J, Poirier J. Alzheimer's disease: current knowledge, management and research. Can Med Assoc J 1997;157:1047–52.

16. Albert SM, Sano M, Marder K, et al. Participation in clinical trials and long-term outcomes in Alzheimer's disease. Neurology 1997;49:38–43.

17. Mittelman MS, Ferris SH, Shulman E, et al. A family intervention to delay nursing home placement of patients with Alzheimer's disease. JAMA 1996;276:1725–31.

18. Beatty WW, Winn P, Adams RL, et al. Preserved cognitive skills in dementia of the Alzheimer type. Arch Neurol 1994;51:1040–6.

Index